Treating the Whole Patient:
Exploring the Healing Potential
of a Mind-Body Approach to
Mental Health

Jon W. Draud, MS, MD
Rakesh Jain, MD, MPH
Vladimir Maletic, MS, MD
Charles Raison, MD

disclaimer

This publication is a compilation of previously posted online blog posts on the community forum for CME LLC's *Treating the Whole Patient* educational initiative.

The opinions and recommendations expressed by the authors and other experts whose input is included in this publication are their own and do not necessarily reflect the views of CME LLC. Discussions concerning drugs, dosages, and procedures may reflect the clinical experience of the authors or may be derived from professional literature or other sources and may suggest uses that are investigational in nature and not approved labeling or indications.

Due to advances in medicine, available clinical data and the potential for human error, the authors and CME LLC do not guarantee that the content is totally accurate or current at the time of reading.

Readers are encouraged to refer to primary references or full prescribing information resources.

about this book

Treating the Whole Patient: Exploring the Healing Potential of a Mind-Body Approach to Mental Health promotes a shift in patient care that encourages healthcare professionals to move beyond a one-dimensional approach to the management of a disease toward a multi-dimensional approach that incorporates new scientific understandings of the many connections between mind and body relevant to diagnosing, treating, and managing patients with psychiatric disorders. Our ultimate goal is to provide an understanding of the neurobiology of a disease and its effect on a patient, consider the role of medical comorbidities on the psychiatric disorder, learn strategies for successful treatment and management options, address barriers to care, and better comprehend the impact of wellness on mental health.

Based on cutting-edge scientific data in fields as diverse as neuroscience, genetics and immunology, *Treating the Whole Patient: Exploring the Healing Potential of a Mind-Body Approach to Mental Health* demonstrate through a question and answer format how recent discoveries promote an integrated mind-body perspective on psychiatric illness that will empower healthcare professionals to optimize therapeutic outcomes by improving multiple aspects of patient care with the long-term result of helping individuals suffering from psychiatric disease to attain wellness.

The *Treating the Whole Patient* mental health initiatives are provided by CME LLC and encompass not only the ongoing community forum of blog posts but also live regional meetings as well as a series of educational sessions at the annual *U.S. Psychiatric and Mental Health Congress*. To view new blogs on this emerging approach to mental health care or find out more information on these initiatives, visit www.cmellc.com/Home/TreatingtheWholePatient.

contents

preface

It is a pleasure to represent my colleagues Drs. Rakesh Jain, Vladimir Maletic, and Charles Raison in writing a brief introduction to our "blog book." As a bit of perspective, we have lectured and traveled widely over the past decade trying to disseminate the basic principles of the neurobiologic underpinnings of neuropsychiatric illnesses. These concepts have evolved to be termed by some as "Mind-Body Science," which have now given a new life to our understanding of the various conditions that affect our patients. This evolving science has also allowed us to explain the conditions in a more mechanistic way that seems to resonate with both physicians and mental health-care providers and patients alike.

This book begins with a manifesto of sorts that calls us to examine psychiatric illness in a radically different way and then, via individual "blog posts," examines the basic neurobiology of certain neuropsychiatric disorders. We continue by providing a discussion of various neuro-endocrine and neuro-immune dysregulations that seem to be common among "stress-related" illnesses including a discussion of the comorbid medical conditions that seem to stem from this mind-body dysregulation. There are chapters related to integrating these concepts and thinking about treatment in new ways, along with several posts on diet, nutrition, and wellness. We include a collection of posts in a chapter on the "Thought and Mood Disorders Continuum" which has become a very hot topic in our field.

Please note that this book is a collection of blogs compiled over two years and is not meant to be a comprehensive treatise on the concepts or topics. By the nature of the book, it begs for a second addition; and by the nature of the topics, the data and ideas are constantly evolving.

We invite you to challenge yourselves with this collection of ideas and stay-tuned for future efforts.

Jon W. Draud, MS, MD

Chapter 1

NEUROBIOLOGY OF PSYCHIATRIC DISORDERS:
IMPLICATIONS FOR TREATING THE WHOLE PATIENT

FROM CHAOS TO CONSILIENCE: PART I

Using the New Mind-Body Science to Improve the Diagnosis and Treatment of Major Depression

Charles Raison, MD, Rakesh Jain, MD, MPH, Vladimir Maletic, MS, MD, and Jon W. Draud, MS, MD:

> **Chaos** – *definition [from wordnet.princeton.edu]: a state of extreme disorder or confusion*
>
> **Consilience** – *definition [from Wikipedia]: literally a jumping together of knowledge by the linking of facts and fact-based theory across disciplines to create a common groundwork for*

Lecturing around the country has left us with the powerful impression that both primary care physicians and psychiatrists are hungry for new ways to think about and manage depression and the myriad symptoms and syndromes with which it is associated—including attention-deficit disorder, insomnia, chronic pain conditions, substance abuse, and various states of disabling anxiety. Primary care physicians also seem especially excited to learn that depression is not just a psychiatric illness, but a behavioral manifestation of underlying pathophysiological processes that promote most of the other conditions they struggle to treat—including cardiovascular disease, diabetes, cancer, and dementia.[1,2]

In hopes of simultaneously quelling and stimulating this hunger and excitement, we have developed a 3-part series that sets forth a new view of major depression that synthesizes multiple converging lines of scientific evidence from an array of fields relevant to mind-body neurobiology. While this new science is fascinating in its own right, our emphasis in this series is to clearly enunciate the promise these new findings hold for improving our ability to diagnose and treat depression and its many comorbidities. We also hope to show that an integrated mind-body view of depression helps explain many aspects of mood disorders that have long been enigmatic. We believe this view can enhance our ability to provide our patients with an honest prognosis for their long-term functioning and survival.

You will find the first article in our series online at www.psychiatrictimes.com. We begin the series with a general discussion of how a mind-body neurobiological approach to depression is an improvement over our current diagnostic understanding of mood and related disorders.

In Part 2, we will detail the primary elements of a mind-body view of depression. In Part 3, we will describe treatment implications that arise from the new science. Throughout, we will highlight ways in which a neurobiological under-standing of mood disorders can help us move toward a personalized approach to the treatment of depression and its multiple comorbidities, both psychiatric and medical.

REFERENCES
1. Miller AH, Maletic V, Raison CL. Inflammation and its discontents: the role of cytokines in the patho-physiology of major depression. *Biol Psychiatry.* 2009;65:732-741.
2. Anand P, Thomas SG, Kunnumakkara AB, et al. Biological activities of curcumin and its analogues (Congeners) made by man and Mother Nature. *Biochem Pharmacol.* 2008;76:1590-1611.

Reprinted with permission from *Psychiatric Times* from Raison CL, Jain R, Maletic V, Draud JW. From chaos to consilience: using the new mind-body science to improve the diagnosis and treatment of major depres-sion. *Psychiatric Times.* 2009;26(5):9.

FROM CHAOS TO CONSILIENCE: PART II

What the New Mind-Body Science Tells Us About the Pathophysiology of Major Depression

Charles Raison, MD, Vladimir Maletic, MS, MD, Rakesh Jain, MD, MPH, and Jon W. Draud, MS, MD:

We would suggest that psychiatry has spent so many years taking its diagnostic categories as God-given that it has become inured to the fact that these categories tell us very little about the etiology and fundamental nature of the conditions they purport to encompass.[1]

Nowhere is this truer than in the case of depression. While the *Diagnostic and Statistical Manual of Mental Disorders* (*DSM*)—like all mythopoetic creations—has been forced to grapple with the complexities of reality by creating an ever larger cast of characters related to one another in ever more complicated ways, the types of deep, consilient understandings of depression that would unify rather than splinter, and that would empower rather than enfeeble, our therapeutic efforts have been consigned to the province of future science.

In this—the second installment in our series on mind-body approaches to mood disorders—we suggest that the future is now. Although we are far, indeed, from a full understanding of all the intricacies of depression, scientific advances during the past decade in fields ranging from immunology to evolutionary biology already provide the outlines for a theory of depression that is consistent, inclusive, and (most important) provides intellectually satisfying and testable answers to many basic questions in front of which the *DSM* must raise a finger to its lips in silence.

Because of space constraints, we can provide only the barest overview of this theory here. We invite you to log on to www.psychiatrictimes.com for a longer and more rigorous discussion of these ideas.

What is depression?

All over the world, depression is the most common emotional/behavioral breakdown pathway for human beings in response to environmental adversity. It is highly stereotyped but also irreducibly probabilistic.[2] It is how humans tend to feel and behave when the internal or external environment seems unmanageably threatening. Tethered to systems necessary for survival, depression is a tendency and a vulnerability, an Achilles heel of hominid evolution.

Recent data increasingly suggest that depression is an emotional/behavioral manifestation of hyperactivity in brain-body systems that evolved to cope with danger and to adapt to changing environmental demands.[3-10] Hyperactivity in these systems is linked to—and perhaps causes—reductions in the activity of central nervous system (CNS) pleasure/novelty and executive decision-making circuitry.[11,12] Across human evolution, these "danger pathways" have been most often activated by psychosocial struggles and by pathogen invasion, which goes far toward explaining why psychosocial stress and sickness are the two primary environmental risk factors for depression.

Why does depression have the symptoms it does?

The short answer is that depression looks so much like a combination of terrible stress and physical illnesses because, in our view, it is essentially a disorder of pathways in the brain and body that evolved to cope with stress and infection, and that produce depressive symptoms when chronically hyperactive.[3,5,6,13] Strong support for this idea comes from studies showing that when bidirectional stress—inflammatory danger pathways are chronically activated—such as occurs during treatment with the cytokine interferon-alpha—most people become depressed or, if not depressed, then exhausted, achy, and upset.[14,15] Conversely, interrupt hyperactivity in key stress-related brain regions, such as the subgenual anterior cingulate, and many profoundly depressed patients have an immediate surcease of their internal torture.[16] Recent data also demonstrate that stimulating activity in cortical areas that suppress stress pathway activity, such as the dorsolateral prefrontal cortex, also leads to profound and rapid improvements in depression.[17]

Consider a young mammal separated from its mother. First comes the terror—the wailing and the calling out. And then, with time, a strange thing happens. The little animal grows silent, dull, and perfectly still. This all makes eminent sense: scream out when there is hope of rescue, but conserve energy and hide from predators when the time for hope has passed.

Depression is an analogue of this phenomenon, which should come as no surprise given its evolutionary origins. Thus, in addition to the anxiety, fear, and internal pain produced by danger pathway activation/dysregulation, depression is also characterized by a loss of pleasure that can be profound. This reflects the fact that in addition to danger pathway activation, depression is typically associated with hypoactivity in "pleasure pathways" running from midbrain into anterior areas of the basal ganglia (i.e., nucleus accumbens). Not surprisingly, many recent studies show that chronic activation of danger pathways—such as the innate immune inflammatory system—compromises dopaminergic signaling in pleasure pathways.[18]

Why are the genes for depression so common?

Short answer: Because genes identified thus far that increase the risk of depression are not depression genes per se, but rather play more general roles in regulating systems that are responsible for multiple physiological functions essential for survival and reproduction. In general, they are genes for operating and regulating danger/adaptation/pleasure pathways in the brain and body. Most often, risk alleles for depression increase/dysregulate activity in danger pathways and/or reduce activity in pleasure and executive pathways in the face of environmental adversity.[19,20] In good times or when exposed to supportive early environments, these alleles contribute to individuals who are perhaps more successful and happier than most.[21-23] Even in bad times, these genes probably promote reproductive success by engendering creativity and intelligence[24]—how else could they survive the threshing of natural selection if they did not confer occasional high pay-off selective advantages to counter their more frequent detrimental effects?

Nonetheless, these ideas are not settled science, and alternative views exist about potential adaptive advantages of depression or even whether genes that promote depression must confer some type of adaptive advantage to be retained in the human genome. Although genes that are specific for depression or that always cause depression regardless of environmental conditions have yet to be identified, this does not prove that such genes may not yet await discovery. If such genes were ever found, it would be expected that they would be very powerful, but also very rare, and therefore would account for only a tiny fraction of individuals with depression.

Would it surprise you to learn that genes reported to increase the risk of developing depression in the face of psychosocial stress also seem to increase the risk of depression in the context of sickness?[25,26] Would you predict that these risk alleles might enhance survival in the face of infection early in life, and that this might also account for their high prevalence in the human gene pool?[27]

Why is depression a risk factor for other diseases and why is it progressive?

While these seem like separate questions, the new mind-body science suggests that they are actually variations on a theme. Depression, in our view, is linked to most other modern illnesses because it shares an underlying pathophysiology with them.[18,28] Millions of years of evolution favored the development and retention of extremely robust stress and inflammatory danger pathways. When death and destruction lurked around every corner, the safest policy was to fire off one's danger pathways first and ask questions later. What did it matter if body and brain tissues were damaged a little each time these pathways activated if this kept one alive for today (an idea that has been popularized as allostatic load).[29] No need to worry about heart disease, cancer, or dementia if you were likely to die of infection by age 30.

Consider our plight today, however. The boss no longer rips your arm off when he shouts at you, and many of the jobs once done by inflammation have been farmed out to sanitation and modern medicine. But the old danger pathways just go on firing off every time someone looks at us sideways. The more they fire off, the more damage accumulates. When this occurs in the arteries, it is vascular disease[30]; when it promotes insulin resistance, it is diabetes[30]; and when it disrupts glial cell integrity and disorganizes neuronal signaling, it manifests as depression.[31,32] Given enough time, the damage usually accumulates everywhere—hence, the high comorbidity between depression and most other major modern maladies.

Why is remission so important?

The new mind-body science suggests that depressive symptoms are a "shout out" that the brain and body are in a state that is inimical to optimal functioning and health in the modern world. Conversely, an implication of the ideas presented here is that depressive symptoms are not likely to improve unless a person's underlying danger pathway functioning normalizes, at least to some degree.[28,33] So remission is the best indicator we currently have that a person's underlying physiology has returned to a safer state. Of course, symptoms are not perfect. If they were, remission would heal all ills.[34] In fact, we know that even when remission is achieved, patients remain at greatly increased risk for sinking again into depression when compared with those who have never suffered depression.[35]

Join us as we next apply the implications of recent scientific advances to the practicalities of diagnosing and treating depression.

REFERENCES

1. First MB. Changes in psychiatric diagnosis. *Psychiatric Times.* 2008;25(13):14-16.
2. Simon GE, VonKorff M, Piccinelli M, et al. An international study of the relation between somatic symptoms and depression. *N Engl J Med.* 1999;341:1329-1335.
3. Raison CL, Capuron L, Miller AH. Cytokines sing the blues: inflammation and the pathogenesis of major depression. *Trends Immunol.* 2006;27:24-31.
4. McEwen BS. Mood disorders and allostatic load. *Biol Psychiatry.* 2003;54:200-207.
5. Maier SF, Watkins LR. Cytokines for psychologists: implications of bidirectional immune-to-brain communication for understanding behavior, mood, and cognition. *Psychol Rev.* 1998;105:83-107.
6. Chen CH, Ridler K, Suckling J, et al. Brain imaging correlates of depressive symptom severity and predictors of symptom improvement after antidepressant treatment. *Biol Psychiatry.* 2007;62:407-414.
7. Siegle GJ, Carter CS, Thase ME. Use of FMRI to predict recovery from unipolar depression with cognitive behavior therapy. *Am J Psychiatry.* 2006;163:735-738.
8. Fitzgerald PB, Laird AR, Maller J, Daskalakis ZJ. A meta-analytic study of changes in brain activation in depression. *Hum Brain Mapp.* 2008;29:683-695.
9. Howren MB, Lamkin DM, Suls J. Associations of depression with C-reactive protein, IL-1, and IL-6: a meta-analysis. *Psychosom Med.* 2009;71:171-186.
10. Pace TW, Mletzko TC, Alagbe O, et al. Increased stress-induced inflammatory responses in male patients with major depression and increased early life stress. *Am J Psychiatry.* 2006;163:1630-1633.
11. Epstein J, Pan H, Kocsis JH, et al. Lack of ventral striatal response to positive stimuli in depressed versus normal subjects. *Am J Psychiatry.* 2006;163: 1784-1790.
12. Siegle GJ, Thompson W, Carter CS, et al. Increased amygdala and decreased dorsolateral prefrontal BOLD responses in unipolar depression: related and independent features. *Biol Psychiatry.* 2007;61:198-209.
13. Dantzer R, O'Connor JC, Freund GG, et al. From inflammation to sickness and depression: when the immune system subjugates the brain. *Nat Rev Neurosci.* 2008;9:46-56.
14. Raison CL, Demetrashvili M, Capuron L, Miller AH. Neuropsychiatric adverse effects of interferon-alpha: recognition and management. *CNS Drugs.* 2005;19: 105-123.
15. Capuron L, Gumnick JF, Musselman DL, et al. Neurobehavioral effects of interferon-alpha in cancer patients: phenomenology and paroxetine responsiveness of symptom dimensions. *Neuropsychopharmacology.* 2002;26:643-652.
16. Mayberg HS. Targeted electrode-based modulation of neural circuits for depression. *J Clin Invest.* 2009;119:717-725.
17. Bares M, Kopecek M, Novak T, et al. Low frequency (1-Hz), right prefrontal repetitive transcranial magnetic stimulation (rTMS) compared with venlafaxine ER in the treatment of resistant depression: a double-blind, single-centre, randomized study. *J Affect Disord.* 2009 Feb 25. [Epub ahead of print.]
18. Miller AH, Maletic V, Raison CL. Inflammation and its discontents: the role of cytokines in the pathophysiology of major depression. *Biol Psychiatry.* 2009;65:732-741.

19. Su S, Miller AH, Snieder H, et al. Common genetic contributions to depressive symptoms and inflammatory markers in middle-aged men: the Twins Heart Study. *Psychosom Med.* 2009;71:152-158.
20. Schule C, Zill P, Baghai TC, et al. Brain-derived neurotrophic factor Val66Met polymorphism and dexamethasone/CRH test results in depressed patients. *Psychoneuroendocrinology.* 2006;31:1019-1025.
21. Kendler KS, Kuhn JW, Vittum J, et al. The interaction of stressful life events and a serotonin transporter polymorphism in the prediction of episodes of major depression: a replication. *Arch Gen Psychiatry.* 2005; 62:529-535.
22. Caspi A, Sugden K, Moffitt TE, et al. Influence of life stress on depression: moderation by a polymorphism in the 5-HTT gene. *Science.* 2003;301:386-389.
23. Pauli-Pott U, Friedl S, Hinney A, Hebebrand J. Serotonin transporter gene polymorphism (5-HTTLPR), environmental conditions, and developing negative emotionality and fear in early childhood. *J Neural Transm.* 2009;116:503-512.
24. Jamison KR. *Touched With Fire: Manic-Depressive Illness and the Artistic Temperament.* New York: Free Press; 1993.
25. Bull SJ, Huezo-Diaz P, Binder EB, et al. Functional polymorphisms in the interleukin-6 and serotonin transporter genes, and depression and fatigue induced by interferon-alpha and ribavirin treatment. *Mol Psychiatry.* 2008 May 6. [Epub ahead of print.]
26. Kraus MR, Al-Taie O, Schafer A, et al. Serotonin-1A receptor gene HTR1A variation predicts interferon-induced depression in chronic hepatitis C. *Gastroenterology.* 2007;132:1279-1286.
27. Gentile DA, Doyle WJ, Zeevi A, et al. Cytokine gene polymorphisms moderate illness severity in infants with respiratory syncytial virus infection. *Hum Immunol.* 2003;64:338-344.
28. Maletic V, Raison CL. Neurobiology of depression, fibromyalgia and neuropathic pain. *Front Biosci.* 2009;14:5291-5338.
29. McEwen BS. Protection and damage from acute and chronic stress: allostasis and allostatic overload and relevance to the pathophysiology of psychiatric disorders. *Ann N Y Acad Sci.* 2004;1032:1-7.
30. Ridker PM. Inflammatory biomarkers and risks of myocardial infarction, stroke, diabetes, and total mortality: implications for longevity. *Nutr Rev.* 2007;65(12, pt 2):S253-S259.
31. McNally L, Bhagwagar Z, Hannestad J. Inflammation, glutamate, and glia in depression: a literature review. *CNS Spectr.* 2008;13:501-510.
32. Rajkowska G, Miguel-Hidalgo JJ. Gliogenesis and glial pathology in depression. *CNS Neurol Disord Drug Targets.* 2007;6:219-233.
33. Ising M, Horstmann S, Kloiber S, et al. Combined dexamethasone/corticotropin releasing hormone test predicts treatment response in major depression—a potential biomarker? *Biol Psychiatry.* 2007;62:47-54.
34. Aubry JM, Gervasoni N, Osiek C, et al. The DEX/CRH neuroendocrine test and the prediction of depressive relapse in remitted depressed outpatients. *J Psychiatr Res.* 2007;41:290-294.
35. Judd LL, Akiskal HS, Maser JD, et al. Major depressive disorder: a prospective study of residual subthreshold depressive symptoms as predictor of rapid relapse. *J Affect Disord.* 1998;50:97-108.

Reprinted with permission from *Psychiatric Times* from Raison CL, Maletic V, Jain R, Draud JW. From chaos to consilience: Part II. *Psychiatric Times.* 2009;26(7):15-21.

FROM CHAOS TO CONSILIENCE: PART III

What the New Mind-Body Science Tells Us About the Pathophysiology of Major Depression—Focus on Treatment

Charles Raison, MD, Rakesh Jain, MD, MPH, Vladimir Maletic, MS, MD, and Jon W. Draud, MS, MD:

Because you are unlikely to die young of wounding or infection, you will almost certainly succumb instead to the ravages of time, delivered—paradoxically enough—by the very "danger" systems that evolved to protect us from the predators and pathogens that—until recently—stole away most of humanity's finest in the first flower of youth.[1]

In a world of predators and pathogens, it was a fair trade-off. The long-term damage to body tissues that ensued from each episode of danger pathway activation was more than recompensed by an increase in short-term survival.[2] Who cared whether oxidative stress from repeated danger pathway activation led to cardiovascular disease at 65 or to dementia at 80 if it saved you from death by infection repeatedly at 10 or 20 or 30? But what about a world in which predators teeter at extinction's edge and pathogens are (at least for now) beaten back by sanitation, public health, and antibiotics—a world in which danger pathway activation is more likely to occur in response to a yellow light than yellow fever?

The central argument in our series of articles is that depression and related diagnostic conditions (e.g., generalized anxiety, social anxiety, posttraumatic stress disorder, bipolar disorder) are characterized by—and frequently result from—chronic hyperactivity/dysregulation of CNS and peripheral danger pathways in response to conditions in the modern world for which this activity is of little, or no, value.[3] Chief among the danger pathways are the hypothalamic-pituitary-adrenal axis, autonomic nervous system (ANS), and innate immune inflammatory response, as well as CNS circuits that activate, modulate, and down-regulate these pathways—including many prefrontal, paralimbic, and limbic cortical regions.

Significant data demonstrate that depression is characterized in the CNS by reductions in prefrontal executive network activity and increases in fight-flight–related limbic and paralimbic activity.[4] In the periphery, depression is characterized by reduced cortisol signaling and parasympathetic activity and by increased sympathetic and inflammatory activation.[5]

The surest way to help our patients is to set remission up as the guiding star toward which our efforts strive. If our patients approach this goal, we are moving in the right direction, no matter what intervention we are employing.

This pattern of abnormality results from complex interactions between multiple "vulnerability" genes and environmental adversity. We put quotation marks around vulnerability because, by contributing to the regulation of danger pathway activity, these genes play essential roles in maintaining physiological homeostasis necessary for survival. Indeed, in the context of health, these genes contribute to the ability of danger pathways to activate regulatory feedback loops (e.g., cortisol is both a stress and anti-stress hormone) that help craft responses to the actual needs of the current environment. However, when overwhelmed by stress or disease, vulnerability genes tend to promote multilevel disruptions in the functioning of this regulatory circuitry. When this occurs in the CNS, inadequate neurotrophic support leads to impaired neuroplasticity in key danger pathway regulatory areas (i.e., hippocampus, prefrontal cortex), which interferes with limbic-paralimbic-cortical processing necessary to restrain ANS and inflammatory activity and to maintain sufficient cortisol signaling. (For a complete discussion of these issues, please see Maletic and Raison.[6])

Depressive symptoms are the most common manifestations of this pattern of danger pathway dysregulation. However, many other modern diseases (cardiovascular disease, diabetes, dementia, cancer) and emotions (loneliness, chronic stress) share this pattern,[7-14] which almost certainly accounts for the multiple lines of comorbidity between sickness, stress, and depression.

But so what?

Any scientific theory worth its salt should be able to make falsifiable predictions about matters of importance. In the case of mental illness, nothing is more important than treatment, so here, in the final installment of this series, we'd like to give a sense of how emerging mind-body understandings can benefit our patients now, and will further benefit them with the development of new treatments.[1]

Of the many hypotheses that are suggested by a mind-body perspective, we offer three here that we feel are especially relevant.

1. *Anything that turns down danger system activity and/or corrects insufficient cortisol signaling should be of benefit for depression.*

To discuss this hypothesis in a manageable fashion, let's focus primarily on inflammation as an example of a danger pathway that is hyperactive in the context of depression. It is a clear prediction of a danger system view of depression that anything that reduces inflammation should be a useful addition to our current treatment armamentarium. For years, people would respond to our talks with a very obvious question, "So why doesn't aspirin work for depression?"

Well, in fact, recent data—although preliminary—suggest that aspirin might indeed have antidepressant properties, on the basis of data showing that the addition of aspirin to fluoxetine converts nonresponders to responders.[15] These findings are in keeping with studies showing that COX-2 inhibitors augment antidepressants in medically healthy patients with major depression.[16,17] Finally, several studies show that cytokine antagonists (which are powerfully anti-inflammatory) diminish depressive symptoms independently of their effects on primary disease processes in patients with autoimmune disorders.[18,19]

While the use of anti-inflammatory agents for medically healthy depressed individuals is not yet quite ready for prime time, a mind-body perspective suggests that strategies currently in use for depression should include anti-inflammatory agents. Indeed this appears to be the case. Multiple studies suggest that both pharmacological and somatic (i.e., electroconvulsive therapy [ECT]) treatments reduce inflammatory biomarkers in medically healthy depressed patients and that these reductions correlate with clinical effect.[20] Recently, cognitive-behavioral therapy has also been shown to reduce inflammation,[21] and compassion meditation has been found to reduce inflammatory responses to stress.[22] Other effective interventions—from exercise and diet to getting enough sleep—also reduce inflammation.[23-25]

Given recent interest in glucocorticoid antagonists for depression,[26] it is an especially germane prediction of our model that these medications will not be shown to be effective for depression or, if they are effective, that they will actually enhance, rather than antagonize, cortisol signaling.[27] (In fact, recent studies are mixed in terms of effectiveness for psychotic depression,[28,29] with no effect being observed for depressive symptoms.[28]) The model also predicts that strategies for reducing sympathetic activity and/or increasing parasympathetic activity should help to ameliorate depression and related conditions. Recent studies suggest that biofeedback methods that accomplish this improve symptoms in depression, in posttraumatic stress disorder, and also in patients who have fibromyalgia.[30-33]

2. Because depression and other modern illnesses are linked via danger pathway hyperactivity, things that are good for depression should be good for your health, and things that are good for your health should be good for depression.

There are so many obvious ways in which these hypotheses are true that we hesitated to include this point, but the topic is so important that we feel it deserves emphasis. If you went to a cardiologist and asked for a list of recommendations for being heart-healthy, what response would you expect? Exercise, meditate, eat an anti-inflammatory diet (i.e., Mediterranean diet), maintain a normal weight, and reduce your stress. A better lifestyle prescription for preventing and/or treating depression couldn't be found. Many studies show that exercise elevates mood and treats depression, and an emerging literature points to the usefulness of meditation for psychological disturbance.[34,35]

Diets rich in omega-3 fatty acids are associated with reduced depression,[36] and diets high in processed sugar are associated with increased depression.[37] (Of course, association does not prove causality; for example, depressed persons may turn to sugar as "self-medication.") Obesity predicts the development of depression[38] and is associated with nonresponse to antidepressant therapy.[39] Disturbingly, recent evidence suggests that obesity may be independently associated with the types of reduction in cerebral gray matter volume that are also seen in depressed persons.[40]

A more controversial, but unequivocal, prediction is that antidepressants and psychotherapy should improve medical illnesses characterized by danger pathway activation. Although not completely concordant, at least some studies suggest that antidepressants protect against or reduce morbidity and/or mortality from cardiac disease, stroke, and diabetes, and that lithium may protect against dementia.[41-44] However, it is important to recognize that like all medications, antidepressants are not infrequently beset with adverse effects that may counteract beneficial actions. So, for example, negative effects of tricyclic antidepressants on cardiac function may outweigh their benefits, and agents associated with weight gain may ramp up danger pathway activity via this mechanism in ways that obviate such effects as anti-inflammatory activity. Again, although the data are mixed, at least some studies suggest that psychotherapy may extend survival in the context of cancer,[45] and a recent meta-analysis indicates that psychological interventions reduce mortality in men with heart disease.[46]

Conversely (and as already suggested), medications that treat medical illnesses by reducing danger pathway activity should also be good for preventing and/or treating depression, even if they are not currently on our radar screen for this indication. Statins are especially intriguing in this regard. Although originally administered to improve lipid status, it is now clear that anti-inflammatory properties are central to their beneficial vascular effects.[47] Because inflammatory processes are increasingly implicated in depression, one would predict that statins should function—at least to some degree—as antidepressants, and indeed data suggest that these agents enhance positive mood and diminish negative mood.[48] Lacking a danger pathway view of depression, these findings might be regarded as curious oddities. With such a view, they make eminent sense and point to the possibility that other medications currently in use for wear-and-tear disorders may hold promise in the treatment of depression.

3a. *Because symptoms emerge probabilistically from danger pathway hyperactivity/dysregulation, similar patterns of physiological activity should give rise to an array of behavioral disturbances currently classified as separate disorders, and individuals at risk for dysregulated danger pathway activity should manifest different patterns of symptoms at different times and/or meet multiple Diagnostic and Statistical Manual of Mental Disorders (DSM) diagnoses concurrently.*

3b. *At the end of the day, putting the full range of specific symptoms that any given patient has into remission is the best guarantee that appropriate physiological functioning has been restored.*

Unfortunately, for any illusions we may have of being on the cutting edge in this article, the truth of hypothesis 3a is hardly controversial. Multiple studies show that genes and environmental factors that increase the risk of depression also increase the risk of many other psychiatric conditions. Similarly, although much has been written about danger pathway dysregulation in depression (e.g., reduced cortisol signaling and increased inflammation), these abnormalities have been observed in an array of conditions—from fibromyalgia to mania.[6,49] That *DSM* psychiatric disorders are highly comorbid goes without saying. So, while not exposing novel truths, a danger pathway understanding of depression provides a coherent framework for understanding why things are the way they are in the world of psychiatry. Contrast this with the current (but disintegrating) dogma that each psychiatric condition is a separate disease with a unique cause. If this were true, why do psychiatric diagnoses so often co-occur, and why do they share so much pathophysiology?

Hypothesis 3b points to a delicious paradox inherent in the mind-body view of depression we espouse. Despite its vulnerability to criticism for being overly general (i.e., explains all psychiatric phenomena on the basis of several simple postulates), a major implication of this theory is that psychiatric generalities (i.e., diagnoses) don't really exist. They are categorical descriptions for nondiscrete and shifting patterns of symptoms—nothing more. Because of this, nothing is more real than the actual symptoms experienced by individual patients sitting in our offices at any given moment. It is the idiosyncratic mélange of symptoms and situations suffered by each patient that must be put right if the well-documented benefits of remission are to be achieved. It is not the diagnoses that go into remission; in the end, it is not even the symptoms. It is the individual in all of his or her unique complexity.

We leave you with a startling implication of this line of thinking. Although symptoms are not perfect guides to the underlying biological abnormalities from which they arise, they are our best guides to the intricate workings of brain and body, given the current limitations of our knowledge. Therefore, anything that leads to the remission of symptoms (and that is not illegal, immoral, or fattening, as one of our fathers used to say) should be in our treatment armamentarium. The surest way to help our patients is to set remission up as the guiding star toward which our efforts strive. If our patients approach this goal, we are moving in the right direction, no matter what intervention we are employing. If they move away from this goal, we need to analyze why and take steps to correct the arc of the patient's emotional/physical life. In a world in which antipsychotics have been shown to work as well as antidepressants for panic disorder,[50] and in which placebo appears to affect the brain in ways similar to active treatments,[51] many of our old certainties are crumbling.

Who are we to say what combination of interventions will heal any given patient? What we can say—on the basis of the new mind-body science—is that, whichever therapeutic pathway we tread with any given individual under our care, is right if it leads to symptomatic remission and a full human life. And it is wrong, or incomplete, if it fails in this regard. When we find the right interventions, we can feel fairly sure that we have brought a patient's underlying danger pathway activity into line with the actual needs of the real world he faces, and that we all share—at least for now.

REFERENCES

1. Westendorp RG. Are we becoming less disposable? *EMBO Rep.* 2004;5:2-6.
2. McEwen BS. Protection and damage from acute and chronic stress: allostasis and allostatic overload and relevance to the pathophysiology of psychiatric disorders. *Ann N Y Acad Sci.* 2004;1032:1-7.
3. Raison CL, Capuron L, Miller AH. Cytokines sing the blues: inflammation and the pathogenesis of major depression. *Trends Immunol.* 2006;27:24-31.
4. Fitzgerald PB, Laird AR, Maller J, Daskalakis ZJ. A meta-analytic study of changes in brain activation in depression [published correction appears in *Hum Brain Mapp.* 2008;29:736]. *Hum Brain Mapp.* 2008;29:683-695.
5. Raison CL, Miller AH. When not enough is too much: the role of insufficient glucocorticoid signaling in the pathophysiology of stress-related disorders. *Am J Psychiatry.* 2003;160:1554-1565.
6. Maletic V, Raison CL. Neurobiology of depression, fibromyalgia and neuropathic pain. *Front Biosci.* 2009;14:5291-5338.
7. Tzoulaki I, Murray GD, Lee AJ, et al. C-reactive protein, interleukin-6, and soluble adhesion molecules as predictors of progressive peripheral atherosclerosis in the general population: Edinburgh Artery Study. *Circulation.* 2005;112:976-983.
8. Pradhan AD, Manson JE, Rifai N, et al. C-reactive protein, interleukin 6, and risk of developing type 2 diabetes mellitus. *JAMA.* 2001;286:327-334.
9. Ridker PM. C-reactive protein and other markers of inflammation in the prediction of cardiovascular disease in women. *N Engl J Med.* 2000;342:836-843.
10. Pyter LM, Pineros V, Galang JA, et al. Peripheral tumors induce depressive-like behaviors and cytokine production and alter hypothalamic-pituitary-adrenal axis regulation. *Proc Natl Acad Sci U S A.* 2009;106:9069-9074.
11. Abercrombie HC, Giese-Davis J, Sephton S, et al. Flattened cortisol rhythms in metastatic breast cancer patients. *Psychoneuroendocrinology.* 2004;29:1082-1092.
12. Kuo HK, Yen CJ, Chang CH, et al. Relation of C-reactive protein to stroke, cognitive disorders, and depression in the general population: systematic review and meta-analysis. *Lancet Neurol.* 2005;4:371-380.
13. Cole SW, Hawkley LC, Arevalo JM, et al. Social regulation of gene expression in human leukocytes. *Genome Biol.* 2007;8:R189.
14. Kiecolt-Glaser JK, Preacher KJ, MacCallum RC, et al. Chronic stress and age-related increases in the proinflammatory cytokine IL-6. *Proc Natl Acad Sci U S A.* 2003;100:9090-9095.
15. Mendlewicz J, Kriwin P, Oswald P, et al. Shortened onset of action of antidepressants in major depression using acetylsalicylic acid augmentation: a pilot open-label study. *Int Clin Psychopharmacol.* 2006;21:227-231.
16. Müller N, Schwarz MJ, Dehning S, et al. The cyclooxygenase-2 inhibitor celecoxib has therapeutic effects in major depression: results of a double-blind, randomized, placebo controlled, add-on pilot study to reboxetine. *Mol Psychiatry.* 2006;11:680-684.
17. Akhondzadeh S, Jafari S, Raisi F, et al. Clinical trial of adjunctive celecoxib treatment in patients with major depression: a double blind and placebo controlled trial. *Depress Anxiety.* 2009;26:607-611.
18. Tyring S, Gottlieb A, Papp K, et al. Etanercept and clinical outcomes, fatigue, and depression in psoriasis: double-blind placebo-controlled randomised phase III trial. *Lancet.* 2006;367:29-35.
19. Persoons P, Vermeire S, Demyttenaere K, et al. The impact of major depressive disorder on the short- and long-term outcome of Crohn's disease treatment with infliximab. *Aliment Pharmacol Ther.* 2005;22:101-110.
20. Miller AH, Maletic V, Raison CL. Inflammation and its discontents: the role of cytokines in the pathophysiology of major depression. *Biol Psychiatry.* 2009;65:732-741.
21. Zautra AJ, Davis MC, Reich JW, et al. Comparison of cognitive behavioral and mindfulness meditation interventions on adaptation to rheumatoid arthritis for patients with and without a history of recurrent depression. *J Consult Clin Psychol.* 2008;76:408-421.
22. Pace TW, Negi LT, Adame DD, et al. Effect of compassion meditation on neuroendocrine, innate im-

mune and behavioral responses to psychosocial stress. *Psychoneuroendocrinology.* 2009;34:87-98.

23. Kohut ML, McCann DA, Russell DW, et al. Aerobic exercise, but not flexibility/resistance exercise, reduces serum IL-18, CRP, and IL-6 independent of beta-blockers, BMI, and psychosocial factors in older adults. *Brain Behav Immun.* 2006;20:201-209.

24. Dai J, Miller AH, Bremner JD, et al. Adherence to the Mediterranean diet is inversely associated with circulating interleukin-6 among middle-aged men: a twin study. *Circulation.* 2008;117:169-175.

25. Irwin MR, Wang M, Ribeiro D, et al. Sleep loss activates cellular inflammatory signaling. *Biol Psychiatry.* 2008;64:538-540.

26. Schatzberg AF, Lindley S. Glucocorticoid antagonists in neuropsychiatric [corrected] disorders [published correction appears in *Eur J Pharmacol.* 2008;592:168]. *Eur J Pharmacol.* 2008;583:358-364.

27. Lewis-Tuffin LJ, Jewell CM, Bienstock RJ, et al. Human glucocorticoid receptor beta binds RU-486 and is transcriptionally active. *Mol Cell Biol.* 2007;27:2266-2282.

28. DeBattista C, Belanoff J, Glass S, et al. Mifepristone versus placebo in the treatment of psychosis in patients with psychotic major depression. *Biol Psychiatry.* 2006;60:1343-1349.

29. Blasey CM, Debattista C, Roe R, et al. A multisite trial of mifepristone for the treatment of psychotic depression: a site-by-treatment interaction. *Contemp Clin Trials.* 2009;30:284-248.

30. Karavidas MK, Lehrer PM, Vaschillo E, et al. Preliminary results of an open label study of heart rate variability biofeedback for the treatment of major depression. *Appl Psychophysiol Biofeedback.* 2007;32:19-30.

31. Hassett AL, Radvanski DC, Vaschillo EG, et al. A pilot study of the efficacy of heart rate variability (HRV) biofeedback in patients with fibromyalgia. *Appl Psychophysiol Biofeedback.* 2007;32:1-10.

32. Zucker TL, Samuelson KW, Muench F, et al. The effects of respiratory sinus arrhythmia biofeedback on heart rate variability and posttraumatic stress disorder symptoms: a pilot study. *Appl Psychophysiol Biofeedback.* 2009;34:135-143.

33. Siepmann M, Aykac V, Unterdorfer J, et al. A pilot study on the effects of heart rate variability biofeedback in patients with depression and in healthy subjects. *Appl Psychophysiol Biofeedback.* 2008;33:195-201.

34. Mead GE, Morley W, Campbell P, et al. Exercise for depression. *Cochrane Database Syst Rev.* 2008;(4):CD004366.

35. Arias AJ, Steinberg K, Banga A, Trestman RL. Systematic review of the efficacy of meditation techniques as treatments for medical illness. *J Altern Complement Med.* 2006;12:817-832.

36. Tanskanen A, Hibbeln JR, Tuomilehto J, et al. Fish consumption and depressive symptoms in the general population in Finland. *Psychiatr Serv.* 2001;52:529-531.

37. Westover AN, Marangell LB. A cross-national relationship between sugar consumption and major depression? *Depress Anxiety.* 2002;16:118-120.

38. Roberts RE, Deleger S, Strawbridge WJ, Kaplan GA. Prospective association between obesity and depression: evidence from the Alameda County Study. *Int J Obes Relat Metab Disord.* 2003;27:514-521.

39. Kloiber S, Ising M, Reppermund S, et al. Overweight and obesity affect treatment response in major depression. *Biol Psychiatry.* 2007;62:321-326.

40. Soreca I, Rosano C, Jennings JR, et al. Gain in adiposity across 15 years is associated with reduced gray matter volume in healthy women. *Psychosom Med.* 2009;71:485-490.

41. Glassman AH, O'Connor CM, Califf RM, et al. Sertraline treatment of major depression in patients with acute MI or unstable angina. *JAMA.* 2002;288:701-709.

42. Robinson RG. Treatment issues in poststroke depression. *Depress Anxiety.* 1998;8(suppl 1):85-90.

43. Abrahamian H, Hofmann P, Prager R, Toplak H. Diabetes mellitus and co-morbid depression: treatment with milnacipran results in significant improvement of both diseases (results from the Austrian MDDM study group). *Neuropsychiatr Dis Treat.* 2009;5:261-266.

44. Yeh HL, Tsai SJ. Lithium may be useful in the prevention of Alzheimer's disease in individuals at risk of presenile familial Alzheimer's disease. *Med Hypotheses.* 2008;71:948-951.

45. Spiegel D, Giese-Davis J. Depression and cancer: mechanisms and disease progression. *Biol Psychiatry.* 2003;54:269-282.

46. Linden W, Phillips MJ, Leclerc J. Psychological treatment of cardiac patients: a meta-analysis. *Eur Heart J.* 2007;28:2972-2984.

47. Ridker PM, Cannon CP, Morrow D, et al. C-reactive protein levels and outcomes after statin therapy. *N Engl J Med.* 2005;352:20-28.

48. Young-Xu Y, Chan KA, Liao JK, et al. Long-term statin use and psychological well-being. *J Am Coll*

Cardiol. 2003;42:690-697.

49. Goldstein BI, Kemp DE, Soczynska JK, McIntyre RS. Inflammation and the phenomenology, patho-physiology, comorbidity, and treatment of bipolar disorder: a systematic review of the literature. *J Clin Psychiatry.* 2009 Jun 2; [Epub ahead of print].

50. Prosser JM, Yard S, Steele A, et al. A comparison of low-dose risperidone to paroxetine in the treatment of panic attacks: a randomized, single-blind study. *BMC Psychiatry.* 2009;9:25.

51. Benedetti F, Mayberg HS, Wager TD, et al. Neurobiological mechanisms of the placebo effect. *J Neurosci.* 2005;25:10390-10402.

Reprinted with permission from *Psychiatric Times* from Raison CL, Jain R, Maletic V, Draud JW. From chaos to consilience: Part III. *Psychiatric Times.* 2009;26(8):25-27.

Bridging the Brain to the Body

QUESTION: "Could you please comment on the quote you cited by Dr. Charles Mayo and how the concept of the progressive nature of neuropsychiatric illnesses bridges the brain to the body?"

Jon W. Draud, MS, MD:

This is an excellent question that gets to the heart of our evolving concept of the mind-body science. Dr. Mayo's astute quote was from 1898 and underscores that for over 100 years physicians have suspected a strong link between the brain and the body. The quote reads: "Worry affects the circulation, the heart, the glands, the whole nervous system. I have never known a man who died of overwork, but many who died from doubt." We clearly see that Dr. Mayo was an early adopter of how profoundly disturbances of the mind could impact bodily functions in the periphery. This is particularly salient given that Western medicine has spent years artificially disconnecting psychiatry and the brain from general medicine and the body.

Carney and colleagues[1] showed that depression is an independent risk factor for death in a five-year, follow-up study that examined survival in patients without depression versus patients with depression post-myocardial infarction. The results are impressive and show that the presence of either major or minor depression increases one's risk for all-cause mortality.

The concept of disease state progression and how this fits into the overall mind-body science is explored in several studies. First, Keller and Boland[2] presented clinically compelling data on recurrence of depression becoming increasingly likely with each successive episode over a five-year period. This data is a clinical pearl in my mind, and reminds us as clinicians that a patient's risk of recurrence is 50% after episode 1, 70% after episode 2, and 90% after episode 3. As clinicians, we also know that our patients suffering third and fourth episodes are much more difficult to treat to remission than those presenting with a first episode of depression.

Part of the rationale for this clinical finding is presented in data from Frodl and colleagues.[3] This three-year, prospective study compared healthy controls to patients with major depression. Patients with major depression had significant differences in the volume of gray matter density in several brain regions, including the hippocampus, amygdala, anterior cingulum, and dorsomedial prefrontal cortex. This is very compelling data for us as daily clinicians, and essentially warns us that depression seems to be a disease that results in neuronal degeneration.

There is further evidence of the same basic pattern of brain volume loss in patients with insomnia as well as patients with fibromyalgia. If we examine the data by Riemann et al.,[4] we see that patients with primary insomnia have significant volume loss in both the right and left hippocampus when compared to good sleepers. Kuchinad and colleagues[5] found that patients with fibromyalgia lost 10.5 cm^3 of gray matter annually since the year of their diagnosis. In addition, there seemed to be greater loss related to advancing age of the patients and the time since their diagnosis.

This brings us full circle to Dr. Mayo's observation over 100 years ago, and should serve as a daily reminder to us as clinicians that the mind and body are inextricably linked in our patients. There seems to be increasing evidence that under- or untreated neuropsychiatric illnesses may similarly lead to brain volume reductions in our patients. This should re-awaken us to our mission of aggressively and comprehensively treating these conditions in our patients to help stave off the sequelae.

REFERENCES

1. Carney RM, Freedland KE, Steinmeyer B, et al. Depression and five year survival following acute myocardial infarction: a prospective study. *J Affect Disord*. 2008;109(1-2):133-138.
2. Keller MB, Boland RJ. Implications of failing to achieve successful long-term maintenance treatment of recurrent unipolar major depression. *Biol Psychiatry*. 1998;44(5):348-360.
3. Frodl TS, Koutsouleris N, Bottlender R, et al. Depression-related variation in brain morphology over 3 years: effects of stress? *Arch Gen Psychiatry*. 2008;65(10):1156-1165.
4. Reimann D, Voderholzer U, Spiegelhalder K, et al. Chronic insomnia and MRI-measured hippocampal volumes: a pilot study. *Sleep*. 2007;30(8):955-958.
5. Kuchinad A, Schweinhardt P, Seminowicz DA, et al. Accelerated brain gray matter loss in fibromyalgia patients: premature aging of the brain? *J Neurosci*. 2007;27(15):4004-4007.

The Brain, Depression, and Remission

QUESTION: "I have been reading that depression can be harmful to the brain. Is this true, and is remission protective to the brain?"

Rakesh Jain, MD, MPH:

You are right, there has been a recent explosion of knowledge in the field regarding the adverse effects of major depression on the various structures of the brain. We have long known that major depression hurts psychological well-being and physical health. Now we are realizing there is one more thing to worry about.

That worry is the impact of depression on both the structure and functioning of the brain.

Let's first quickly review the evidence. It appears that major depression is much more than just an "emotional" disorder, because significant biological events occur when someone is "just" depressed. These events include (but are not limited to) hypothalamic-pituitary-adrenal (HPA) axis dysregulation, autonomic dysregulation, neurotrophic dysregulation, and inflammatory cytokine dysregulation.[1,2] All of these factors (and many others we don't yet know about) collude to create structural and functional harm to the brain.[3-6] In and of itself, structural changes are worrisome, but it's the related cognitive-emotional deterioration that makes these issues important to every clinician.[7,8]

The evidence points to altered structures in major depression in several parts of the brain. Most of these structures are in one way or another involved with stress regulation, mood regulation, and/or sleep regulation. The evidence is most striking for hippocampus, amygdala, and prefrontal cortex. Space limits a full discussion of these neurobiological data, but I am providing a few references here that you may wish to review for further clarification.[9-11]

While many studies support this neurodegenerative issue, it's important to point out that not every study reveals this finding—the issue of depression "damaging" the brain is not yet a fully settled one.[12] Another interesting finding is that these structural differences extend to not just patients, but also to individuals who don't have major depression, but have high familial risk factors for depression.[13] This, of course, raises a perennial question: "The chicken or the egg? Which came first?" Does a person get depression first and then suffer the structural damage, or are individuals with smaller brain structures more likely to suffer from depression? The answer appears to be both.

The negative effects of depression on the brain extend beyond major depression. Bipolar depression also appears to have a negative structural impact on the brain.[14] Additionally, having a comorbid medical condition along with major depression may further challenge the structural integrity of the brain.[15]

What are some of the ways to protect the brain? There is good evidence that physical exercise is protective,[16] and, therefore, recommending physical exercise to all patients is good advice for multiple reasons.

Remission in depression does actually appear to protect the brain. Recent, highly influential studies show that, in the long term, remission of symptoms appears protective to the brain.[17-21] Protecting brain volume is obviously important for a multitude of reasons, not the least of which is that increased brain volume predicts positive treatment response.[22,23]

In conclusion, depression is indeed deleterious to the brain. Protecting it appears to be an important goal for a vast number of reasons. Treating depression to remission appears to be one way to reduce the insult to the brain.[24] The take-home message here is quite straightforward to us clinicians, isn't it? Identify and treat depression, and treat it as aggressively as necessary in order to achieve remission.

REFERENCES

1. Dean B, Tawadros N, Scarr E, Gibbons AS. Regionally-specific changes in levels of tumour necrosis factor in the dorsolateral prefrontal cortex obtained postmortem from subjects with major depressive disorder. *J Affect Disord*. 2010;120(1-3):245-248.
2. Maes M, Yirmiya R, Noraberg J, et al. The inflammatory & neurodegenerative (I&ND) hypothesis of depression: leads for future research and new drug developments in depression. *Metab Brain Dis*. 2009;24(1):27-53.
3. Campbell S, Marriott M, Nahmias C, MacQueen GM. Lower hippocampal volume in patients suffering from depression: a meta-analysis. *Am J Psychiatry*. 2004;161(4):598-607.
4. Bremner JD, Vythilingam M, Vermetten E, et al. Deficits in hippocampal and anterior cingulate functioning during verbal declarative memory encoding in midlife major depression. *Am J Psychiatry*. 2004;161(4):637-645.
5. Sheline YI, Mittler BL, Mintun MA. The hippocampus and depression. *Eur Psychiatry*. 2002;17(suppl 3):300-305.
6. Bremner JD. Structural changes in the brain in depression and relationship to symptom recurrence. *CNS Spectr*. 2002;7(2):129-130, 135-139.
7. Drevets WC. Neuroimaging and neuropathological studies of depression: implications for the cognitive-emotional features of mood disorders. *Curr Opin Neurobiol*. 2001;11(2):240-249.
8. Frodl T, Schaub A, Banac S, et al. Reduced hippocampal volume correlates with executive dysfunctioning in major depression. *J Psychiatry Neurosci*. 2006;31(5):316-323.
9. Maletic V, Raison CL. Neurobiology of depression, fibromyalgia and neuropathic pain. *Front Biosci*. 2009;14:5291-5338.
10. Miller AH, Maletic V, Raison CL. Inflammation and its discontents: the role of cytokines in the pathophysiology of major depression. *Biol Psychiatry*. 2009;65(9):732-741.
11. Maletic V, Robinson M, Oakes T, et al. Neurobiology of depression: an integrated view of key findings. *Int J Clin Pract*. 2007;61(12):2030-2040.
12. Koolschijn PC, van Haren NE, Schnack HG, et al. Cortical thickness and voxel-based morphometry in depressed elderly. *Eur Neuropsychopharmacol*. 2010;20(6):398-404.
13. Chen MC, Hamilton JP, Gotlib IH. Decreased hippocampal volume in healthy girls at risk of depression. *Arch Gen Psychiatry*. 2010;67(3):270-276.
14. Brooks JO 3rd, Bonner JC, Rosen AC, et al. Dorsolateral and dorsomedial prefrontal gray matter density changes associated with bipolar depression. *Psychiatry Res*. 2009;172(3):200-204.
15. Kumar A, Gupta R, Thomas A, et al. Focal subcortical biophysical abnormalities in patients diagnosed with type 2 diabetes and depression. *Arch Gen Psychiatry*. 2009;66(3):324-330.
16. Floel A, Ruscheweyh R, Kruger K, et al. Physical activity and memory functions: are neurotrophins and cerebral gray matter volume the missing link? *Neuroimage*. 2010;49(3):2756-2763.
17. Li CT, Lin CP, Chou KH, et al. Structural and cognitive deficits in remitting and non-remitting recurrent depression: a voxel-based morphometric study. *Neuroimage*. 2010;50(1):347-356.
18. Costafreda SG, Chu C, Ashburner J, Fu CH. Prognostic and diagnostic potential of the structural neu-

roanatomy of depression. *PLoS One.* 2009;4(7):e6353.

19. Yucel K, McKinnon M, Chahal R, et al. Increased subgenual prefrontal cortex size in remitted patients with major depressive disorder. *Psychiatry Res.* 2009;173(1):71-76.

20. Lorenzetti V, Allen NB, Whittle S, Yucel M. Amygdala volumes in a sample of current depressed and remitted depressed patients and healthy controls. *J Affect Disord.* 2010;120(1-3):112-119.

21. Frodl T, Meisenzahl EM, Zetzsche T, et al. Hippocampal and amygdala changes in patients with major depressive disorder and healthy controls during a 1-year follow-up. *J Clin Psychiatry.* 2004;65(4):492-499.

22. MacQueen GM, Yucel K, Taylor VH, et al. Posterior hippocampal volumes are associated with remission rates in patients with major depressive disorder. *Biol Psychiatry.* 2008;64(10):880-883.

23. Frodl T, Jager M, Born C, et al. Anterior cingulate cortex does not differ between patients with major depression and healthy controls, but relatively large anterior cingulate cortex predicts a good clinical course. *Psychiatry Res.* 2008;163(1):76-83.

24. Frodl T, Jager M, Smajstrlova I, et al. Effect of hippocampal and amygdala volumes on clinical outcomes in major depression: a 3-year prospective magnetic resonance imaging study. *J Psychiatry Neurosci.* 2008;33(5):423-430.

Genetic Contribution in Major Depressive Disorder

QUESTION: "What is the extent of genetic contribution in MDD? I thought that it was mostly a stress-induced condition."

Vladimir Maletic, MS, MD:

Major depressive disorder (MDD) is believed to be a product of interaction between several vulnerability genes and environmental adversity (this includes stress, trauma, and also medical illness).[1]

There are differing opinions about the relative contribution of genes versus environment. Before one broaches the topic of etiopathogenesis, it would be prudent to clarify the definition of MDD as a diagnostic category. Recent research suggests that MDD is not a single biological entity, but rather a grouping of biologically diverse conditions with similar symptomatic manifestations. Therefore, any statement made about the origins of MDD is by necessity probabilistic: it may apply to a significant number of individuals afflicted by MDD, but certainly not to all of them.[1]

The body of genetic research into origins of MDD would indicate a strong influence of heritability. While estimates of heritability range from 30% to 50%, it is clear that environment has at least an equal, if not greater, contribution.[2] Genetic pattern of MDD inheritance is a very complex one. Vulnerability towards MDD is conferred by interactions of multiple different genes with differing magnitude of effect. Estimates vary from dozens of genes with moderate-to-mild effect on one end, to a cumulative impact of thousands of genes with minor individual contributions at the other extreme. Research into MDD genetics is further confounded by complicated gene interactions (a process also known as epistasis): two "vulnerability" genes may have a synergistic effect, amplifying each other's influence, or their contributions may cancel each other out![1]

Relatively recent research has focused on the influence of epigenetic modulation in etiology of MDD. It appears that our life experiences have a profound impact on regulation of gene expression. Early life experience seems to be particularly influential in this regard. A study by Etringer et al.[3] has found that stressful experiences in pregnancy had a profound effect on a child's hypothalamic-pituitary-adrenal function in a stressful condition, noticeable even two decades later!

REFERENCES
1. Maletic V, Raison CL. Neurobiology of depression, fibromyalgia and neuropathic pain. *Front Biosci.* 2009;14:5291-5318.
2. Merikangas K, Yu K. Genetic epidemiology of bipolar disorder. *Clin Neurosci Res.* 2002;2(3-4):127-141.
3. Entringer S, Kumsta R, Hellhammer DH, et al. Prenatal exposure to maternal psychosocial stress and HPA axis regulation in young adults. *Horm Behav.* 2009;55(2):292-298.

Genetics: Schizophrenia and Major Depressive Disorder

QUESTION: "Is it true that schizophrenia and major depressive disorder have shared genetic underpinning?"

Vladimir Maletic, MS, MD:

Yes, it appears that schizophrenia and major depressive disorder (MDD) have some shared "vulnerability" genes. Before we continue with the discussion of the overlapping genetics of MDD and schizophrenia, it is appropriate to point out that these conditions are a byproduct of an interaction between genetic predilection and environmental adversity. Schizophrenia has higher heritability than MDD (defined as portion of phenotypical variance explained by genetics).[1,2] Heritability estimates are based on identical twin concordance rates: if one of the twins has the condition, what are the odds that the other one will also have it? Heritability estimates for schizophrenia range from 50% to 90%; usually literature quotes 70% as an approximation.[1] Although population-based twin studies place heritability of MDD in the 30% to 40% range, a more methodologically advanced hospital-based study has found MDD heritability in excess of 70%![2,3]

Now may be a good time to mention that "genetics" represent a complex category comprised of several interrelated processes. Genes tend to be organized into so-called "genetic networks," with interdependent activity and products (structural proteins, enzymes, etc.).[3] Genes and their products tend to interact with each other through a process of genetic epistasis, either potentiating or diminishing each other's effects. Activity of the genes can also be altered through epigenetic modulation; they can be either turned "on" by acetylation of the histone or silenced through histone methylation.

Many of the candidate genes for schizophrenia that code for products regulating monoamine signaling (catechol-O-methyltransferase [COMT], monoamine, and tyrosine hydroxylase) are also considered susceptibility genes for MDD.[3,4,5] Monoamines have a major role in modulating gamma-aminobutyric acid (GABA) and glutamate signaling in frontal cortico-limbic circuitry, which is responsible for regulation of executive function, mood, pain, and stress response.[5] Additionally, genes that regulate GABA and glutamate trafficking are also on the candidate list for MDD and schizophrenia.[4,5]

Neuroplasticity allows our brains to "rewire" themselves in response to sustained change in pattern of activity in a part of neural network, often reflecting an important learning or a change in our environment. Neurotrophins, including brain-derived neurotrophic factor (BDNF), are the key regulators of neuroplasticity. Genes coding for BDNF are implicated in both schizophrenia and MDD. In order for neural signaling to flow smoothly, neurons and astroglia cells need to appropriately collaborate with each other. Aside from removing excessive neurotransmitters from the synapse (thus regulating the signal to noise ratio), glia cells also match the blood perfusion rate with the level of synaptic activity, and provide nerve cells with auxiliary energy (lactate) in times of increased need.[5] D-serine is one of the "glia-transmitters" used in the dialogue between glia and nerve cells. It is also an important modifier of N-methyl-D-aspartate (NMDA)-mediated glutamate signaling and, indirectly, neuroplasticity. I think that you have already guessed: it has been identified as one of the genes conferring predilection for both schizophrenia and MDD.[2,4]

In summary, genes that regulate different interlinked aspects of neural function from monoamine regulation to GABA and glutamate signaling, neuroplasticity, and successful neuron-glia dialogue are implicated in both disease states. There are some more unlikely suspects as well: genes involved in immune function and regulation of inflammatory response are also considered as candidate genes in both MDD and schizophrenia.[4,5]

More recent genetic theories have focused on the role of rare copy number variants (CNVs) in pathogenesis of psychiatric illness. Structural variations reflected in loss or gain of millions of base pairs of DNA sequences are believed to represent more than 5% of human genome.[6] Rare CNVs have been identified in patients with schizophrenia, and may be associated with elevated risk in more neurodevelopmental forms of this disease.[6] A better understanding of the role that CNVs play in pathogenesis of psychiatric disorders may shed light on subtypes of conditions and spectrums of disease.

Finally, whether a condition becomes manifest or not may depend on efficient silencing of nuisance genes. We have already identified methylation as an important modifier of gene expression. In order for methylation to proceed smoothly, genes regulating methyl-donor availability need to function properly. Methylenetetrahydrofolate reductase (MTHFR) is a key enzyme determining methyl group availability. Each copy of its genetic 677T variant conveys a 35% reduction in MTHFR activity and, therefore, a lesser ability to silence other pesky genes.[7] Val copy of COMT gene is associated with more efficient breakdown of dopamine and norepinephrine in the prefrontal cortex, and consequently perhaps more vulnerable executive function. It may be advantageous to keep this gene silenced.

Patients with schizophrenia homozygous for the COMT Val allele who were also misfortunate to have a dysfunctional T variant of MTHFR gene predictably performed more poorly on tests of executive function such as Wisconsin Card Sorting Task.[7] In a separate study, TT carriers of MTHFR gene were 22% more likely to have current or a history of depression.[8] Furthermore, a study of pregnant women has found that presence of MTHFR T-variant was correlated with greater severity of depression.[9] A greater degree of maternal depression was also associated with lesser methylation (silencing) of dysfunctional 5HTT (serotonin transporter) genes in both mothers and infants! This concerning turn of events may help us understand how genetic epistasis and epigenetic modulation may play a role in developmental programming of an infant.

REFERENCES

1. Tsuang M. Schizophrenia: genes and environment. *Biol Psychiatry*. 2000;47(3):210-220.
2. McGuffin P, Knight J, Breen G, et al. Whole genome linkage scan of recurrent depressive disorder from the depression network study. *Hum Mol Genet*. 2005;14(22):3337-3345.
3. McGuffin P, Perroud N, Uher R, et al. The genetics of affective disorder and suicide. *Eur Psychiatry*. 2010;25(5):275-277.
4. Sun J, Jia P, Fanous AH, et al. Schizophrenia gene networks and pathways and their applications for novel gene selection. *PLoS One*. 2010;5(6):e11351
5. Maletic V, Raison CL. Neurobiology of depression, fibromyalgia and neuropathic pain. *Front Biosci*. 2009;14:5291-5338.
6. Bassett AS, Scherer SW, Brzustowicz LM. Copy number variations in schizophrenia: critical review and new perspectives on concepts of genetics and disease. *Am J Psychiatry*. 2010;167(8):899-914.
7. Roffman JL, Weiss AP, Deckersbach T, et al. Interactive effects of COMT Val108/158Met and MTHFR C677T on executive function in schizophrenia. *Am J Med Genet B Neuropsychiatr Genet*. 2008;147B(6):990-995.
8. Almeida OP, McCaul K, Hankey GJ, et al. Homocysteine and depression in later life. *Arch Gen Psychiatry*. 2008;65(11):1286-1294.
9. Devlin AM, Brain U, Austin J, Oberlander TF. Prenatal exposure to maternal depressed mood and the MTHFR C677T variant affect SLC6A4 methylation in infants at birth. *PLoS One*. 2010;5(8):e12201.

Epigenetic Modulation and Major Depressive Disorder

QUESTION: "Is there a role for epigenetic modulation in the etiology of major depressive disorder?"

Vladimir Maletic, MS, MD:

Most likely, yes! During the life cycle of the cell, in response to metabolic perturbations or meaningful environmental changes, profound alterations in gene expression take place—epigenetic modification mediates these processes. Epigenetic modulation is a biological underpinning of cell differentiation; it can also be precipitated by significant events in one's life such as abuse, neglect, extreme poverty, and family dysfunction. In some way, regulation of gene expression mirrors our life experience. Dramatic events in our early childhood appear to leave deeper epigenetic "marks" than adverse events taking place later in our lives.[1]

How is it that our gene expression becomes "reprogrammed"? Our genes, built into sections of DNA strand, are enwrapped by a polypeptide "sleeve" composed of histones. Methylation of histone and/or DNA makes them virtually inaccessible for transcription—the gene is silenced! Acetylation of histone facilitates gene transcription; deacetylation turns it off. A very simplified scenario would suggest that major life events, represented by their chemical correlates, alter the molecular milieu surrounding the cells and consequently cause intracellular signaling cascades, ultimately leaving their specific imprint by changing the pattern of gene expression.[2-4]

An intriguing study by Fraga et al. found that due to a divergent pattern of histone acetylation and methylation, thus turning their genes on or off, a pair of identical twins, after several decades, remained identical in name only.[5] A recent preclinical study indicated that mice subjected to chronic and unpredictable maternal separation developed a behavioral pattern reminiscent of depression. Not only did these depressive-like behaviors persist into adulthood, they were propagated to subsequent generations, suggesting that epigenetically acquired traits may be passed on to progeny.[6]

Let's now examine some of the evidence indicating that epigenetic modulation may have a role in etiopathogenesis of major depressive disorder (MDD). A recent human study focusing on epigenetic modification of a serotonin transporter related gene (5HTTLPR) noted that complete or partial methylation of surrounding histone substantially reduced 5-HT activity.[7] This is of particular interest since 5HTT-linked polymorphic region (5-HTTLPR) alleles have been associated with a number of different neuropsychiatric conditions, including depression, bipolar and anxiety disorders, chronic pain, fibromyalgia, attention-deficit/hyperactivity disorder, insomnia, and substance abuse.

Another study assessed depressed mood in a group of women during the second and third trimesters of pregnancy, using the Edinburgh Postnatal Depression Scale (EPDS) and the Hamilton Rating Scale for Depression (HAM-D). The methylation status of 5-HTTLPR and brain-derived neurotrophic factor (BDNF)-related genes was assessed in third trimester maternal peripheral leukocytes and in umbilical cord leukocytes collected from their infants at birth. A gene regulating methyl-tetra-hydro-folate reductase (MTHFR)—an enzyme with a key role in the synthesis of methyl group donors (and therefore influential in epigenetic methylation)—was also studied. Future mothers with the MTHFR 677TT genotype (less functional allele) had greater second trimester depressed mood. Increased second trimester maternal depressed mood (reflected in EPDS scores) was associated with decreased maternal and infant 5-HTT promoter methylation![8] Less functional genetic variant of 5HTT promoter was inadequately silenced. These findings suggest that maternal depression via altered epigenetic processes may contribute to developmental programming of infant behavior in utero.

In a separate study, adoptees now in their late 30s experienced a greater sense of loss and trauma if their less functional 5-HTTLPR "ss" allele was lightly methylated, or conversely, if their high-functioning "l/l" allele was "silenced" by heavy methylation.[9] Maltreatment during childhood was also found to be associated with methylation of a gene regulating synthesis of an important neurotrophic factor (BDNF) in prefrontal cortex (PFC).[10] Diminished BDNF concentration in PFC has been a consistent finding in postmortem studies of patients with depression.

Adults who have experienced adversity in childhood, such as neglect, family violence, or physical and sexual abuse, are much more likely to develop depression in the face of a current stressful event, according to a recent research report.[11] A landmark prospective study evaluated the impact of early-life adversity on the likelihood of developing adult depression and general medical conditions. Adults who suffered adversity in their childhood were much more likely to develop MDD, but also clustering of metabolic and inflammatory markers several decades later! Furthermore, authors reported a "dose-response" relationship between the number of adverse childhood experiences and the likelihood of developing subsequent pathology.[12]

A paper stemming from a prospective National Collaborative Perinatal Project (mean age=34 at follow-up, final N=482) noted an association between objectively measured affective quality of the mother-infant interaction (rated by an observer when infants were eight months old), and adult mental health. Highly affectionate parent-child interaction at the age of eight months was associated with reduced anxiety and somatization in adults (measured by a standardized instrument) three decades later![13]

In summary, accumulating evidence points to a dramatic impact of early-life adversity on the adult mental and even general medical health. Most likely, early events left an epigenetic "imprint" manifest in mind and bodily function decades later. It appears that the same epigenetic processes, which assist with cellular differentiation at the microscopic level, may also play a role in the differentiation of the major bodily regulatory systems, and even personality at the macroscopic level.

REFERENCES
1. Champagne FA, Curley JP. How social experiences influence the brain. *Curr Opin Neurobiol.* 2005;15(6):704-709.
2. Lanzuolo C, Orlando V. The function of the epigenome in cell reprogramming. *Cell Mol Life Sci.* 2007;64(9):1043-1062.
3. McClung CA, Nestler EJ. Neuroplasticity mediated by altered gene expression. *Neuropsychopharmacology.* 2008;33(1):3-17.
4. Mill J, Petronis A. Molecular studies of major depressive disorder: the epigenetic perspective. *Mol Psychiatry.* 2007;12(9):799-814.
5. Fraga MF, Ballestar E, Paz MF, et al. Epigenetic differences arise during the lifetime of monozygotic twins. *Proc Natl Acad Sci U S A.* 2005;102(30):10604-10609.
6. Franklin TB, Russig H, Weiss IC, et al. Epigenetic transmission of the impact of early stress across generations. *Biol Psychiatry.* 2010;68(5):408-415.
7. Olsson CA, Foley DL, Parkinson-Bates M, et al. Prospects for epigenetic research within cohort studies of psychological disorder: a pilot investigation of a peripheral cell marker of epigenetic risk for depression. *Biol Psychol.* 2010;83(2):159-165.
8. Devlin AM, Brain U, Austin J, Oberlander TF. Prenatal exposure to maternal depressed mood and the MTHFR C677T variant affect SLC6A4 methylation in infants at birth. *PLoS One.* 2010;5(8).pii:12201.
9. van IJzendoorn MH, Caspers K, Bakersmans-Kranenburg MJ, et al. Methylation matters: interaction between methylation density and serotonin transporter genotype predicts unresolved loss or trauma. *Biol Psychiatry.* 2010;68(5):405-407.
10. Roth TL, Lubin FD, Funk AJ, Sweatt JD. Lasting epigenetic influence of early-life adversity on the BDNF gene. *Biol Psychiatry.* 2009;65(9):760-769.
11. McLaughlin KA, Conron KJ, Koenen KC, Gilman SE. Childhood adversity, adult stressful life events, and risk of past-year psychiatric disorder: a test of the stress sensitization hypothesis in a population-based sample of adults. *Psychol Med.* 2010;40(10):1647-1658.
12. Danese A, Moffitt TE, Harrington H, et al. Adverse childhood experiences and adult risk factors for age-related disease: depression, inflammation, and clustering of metabolic risk markers. *Arch Pediatr Adolesc Med.* 2009;163(12):1135-1143.
13. Maselko J, Kubzansky L, Lipsitt L, Buka SL. Mother's affection at 8 months predicts emotional distress in adulthood. *J Epidemiol Community Health.* 2010;[Epub ahead of print].

Ventromedial Prefrontal Cortex Activity in Major Depressive Disorder

QUESTION: "Is the increased activity in ventromedial prefrontal cortex (vmPFC) in major depressive disorder (MDD) a function of loss of volume, as an adaptive mechanism, or is it a separate mechanism?"

Vladimir Maletic, MS, MD:

The challenge in answering this question starts with the definition of vmPFC. Some authors define vmPFC as a structure inclusive of Brodmann Area (BA) 11, 25, and 32; others limit it only to 11 and 32. Distinction is relevant because BA 25 is commonly considered to be the subgenual anterior cingulate cortex (sgACC). Although both of these areas have rich bidirectional connections with limbic areas, especially the amygdala, there are also notable functional differences.[1]

sgACC is one of the main recipients of signals from the amygdala. It is involved in motivational processes and continuous monitoring of emotional salience of our adaptive behaviors. If emotional outcomes do not match our expectations, feedback flow will adjust activity of limbic areas and alter our motivational structure. Increased metabolic activity and substantially reduced gray matter volume of sgACC are one of the most consistent findings in MDD. Although initial reports found decreased sgACC metabolic activity in patients with MDD, once corrections were made for loss of gray matter, researchers concluded that activity is elevated (possibly in a compensatory manner). A number of authors attribute impaired emotional regulation, compromised stress response, and diminished motivation to functional and structural abnormalities in this brain region.

Decreased volume of vmPFC (also referred to as medial orbital PFC) has been a frequently replicated finding in MDD.[2]

Functional imaging studies have had diverse outcomes: increased, decreased, and unchanged activity compared to healthy controls. Biological heterogeneity of MDD and methodological differences may account for these discrepant findings. Elevated vmPFC metabolic activity in MDD has been correlated with intensity of sad affect and depressive ruminations. Apparently, increase in vmPFC activity may be a compensatory response, focused on suppression of negative emotions in context of depression. vmPFC may also provide regulatory feedback to amygdala and brainstem autonomic centers modulating sympathetic/parasympathetic balance. Its dysfunction may give rise to dysautonomia, a common feature of MDD.

REFERENCES
1. Drevets WC, Price JL, Furey ML. Brain structural and functional abnormalities in mood disorders: implications for neurocircuitry models of depression. *Brain Struct Funct*. 2008;213(1-2):93-118.
2. Lacerda AL, Keshavan MS, Hardan AY, et al. Anatomic evaluation of the orbitofrontal cortex in major depressive disorder. *Biol Psychiatry*. 2004;55(4):353-358.

Depression and Diminished Capacity for Pleasure

QUESTION: **"Is there any objective neurobiological evidence indicating that depressed patients have diminished capacity for pleasure?"**

Vladimir Maletic, MS, MD:

The short answer is: most likely. In a very simplified view, the "limbic triangle" composed of amygdala, nucleus accumbens/ventral striatum complex, and hippo-campus is involved in providing a running emotional commentary on perpetual changes in our external and internal environment. Amygdala responds to novelty, especially dangerous and threatening signals. In contrast, nucleus accumbens, also a "novelty detector," tends to preferentially respond to joyous, rewarding events. Amygdala and nucleus accumbens compete for hippocampal "attention." After "sifting" through the inputs, hippocampus generates an emotional association re-lated to the recent event that is subsequently stored in contextual memory. This is an ongoing, reiterative process influenced by constant flow of sensory informa-tion from thalamus and integrative cortical areas. If emotions are confusing or incongruent with our expectations, the signal may be forwarded for secondary processing to higher cortical areas. Emotions may be interpreted as an impetus, a homeostatic signal capable of eliciting a suite of adaptive behavioral responses.

In major depressive disorder (MDD), emotions may lose some of their adap-tive value. Individuals with depression become steeped in misery and dejection, often accompanied by morose rumination. Adaptive exchange with our environ-ment is disrupted; depression takes over as the conductor of our limbic orchestra. Thus, our mood state, rather than ongoing interaction with the environment, becomes the principal determinant of our emotions.

Although empirical evidence is not unequivocal, most of the recent studies point to disturbance of cortico-limbic emotional regulation in MDD. Epstein et al.[1] compared activity of ventral striatum/nucleus accumbens (VST/NAC) com-plex to positive, neutral, and negative stimuli in participants with depression ver-sus healthy controls. They found that there was no difference in the VST/NAC response to neutral and negative stimuli in participants with depression relative to healthy controls. By contrast, participants with depression had much attenuated response, in these reward-related areas, to positive verbal cues (words like "heroic" and "successful"). Diminished VST/NAC activation in response to positive cues correlated with decreased interest and ability to experience pleasure in partici-pants with depression.

Other studies have found decreased signal in emotion-regulating anterior cin-gulate areas correlated with the level of anhedonia observed in patients with de-pression.[2] On the other hand, research has established that amygdala response to negatively valenced cues (even the ones outside our conscious perception) tends to be exaggerated in individuals with depression relative to healthy controls.[3,4] Therefore, it appears that experiential bias in individuals with depression, likely due to malfunction of cortico-limbic circuits, tends to interpret the world as a more sad and threatening place, while minimizing the potentially joyous and rewarding aspects of life.

REFERENCES
1. Epstein J, Pan H, Kocsis JH, et al. Lack of ventral striatal response to positive stimuli in depressed versus normal subjects. *Am J Psychiatry*. 2006;163(10):1784-1790.
2. Walter M, Henning A, Grimm S, et al. The relationship between aberrant neuronal activation in the pregenual anterior cingulate, altered glutamatergic metabolism, and anhedonia in major depression. *Arch Gen Psychiatry*. 2009;66(5):478-486.
3. Hooley JM, Gruber SA, Parker HA, et al. Cortico-limbic response to personally challenging emotional stimuli after complete recovery from depression. *Psychiatry Res*. 2009;172(1):83-91.
4. Sheline YI, Barch DM, Donnelly JM, et al. Increased amygdala response to masked emotional faces in depressed subjects resolves with antidepressant treatment: an fMRI study. *Biol Psychiatry*. 2001;50(9):651-658.

The Role of Glia in Major Depressive Disorder, Have We Been Missing it All Along?

QUESTION: "Is it true that glia cells are the primary brain cell group impacted by depression?"

Vladimir Maletic, MS, MD:

We have unjustly neglected the role of glia cells in neuropsychiatric conditions for a long time. Accumulating evidence suggests that glia cells may be implicated in major depressive disorder (MDD)-related pathology.[1-8] The human nervous system has approximately 100 billion neurons and one trillion glia cells, making them an overwhelming majority.

Three families of glia cells have very different roles and histological origin. Astroglia are co-partners with neurons in neural transmission and provide structural support. Oligodendroglia are involved with myelination of white matter tracts connecting various components of brain circuitry. Microglia are the main immune cells of the brain; they are of mesodermal origin, unlike astroglia and oligodendroglia, which are of ectodermal origin.[1,2,8]

Brain architecture appears to be shaped by astrocytes. Each human astrocyte contacts and encapsulates approximately two million synapses! In addition to managing the content of the synaptic cleft, astroglia may have a role in synchronizing the activity of all neurons within their "domains." Brain connectivity is effectively shaped by astroglia through regulation of synaptic plasticity. Evidence suggests that neurotrophic factors, such as brain-derived and glia-derived neurotrophic factors (BDNF and GDNF), are synthesized within glia cells.

Almost all classes of serotonin, norepinephrine, dopamine, cholinergic, gamma-aminobutyric acid (GABA), glutamate, neurotrophin, and cytokine receptors are expressed on glial cell membranes. Additionally, astroglial membranes express monoamine (5-HTT, NAT, DAT) and glutamate transporters. Probably about half of the monoamine uptake sites blocked by conventional antidepressants are located on glia cells![1,2,8]

However, unlike neurons, which release neurotransmitters in response to action potentials, glia cells discharge their transmitters in response to graded increases in cytoplasmic Ca++. "Analog" pattern of glial transmitter release, in contrast to "binary" neuronal transmission, may have contributed to our long-standing neglect of the astroglial role in neural signaling.[8]

Astroglia also have a role in regulating neuronal energy supply: at times of peak neuronal activity, glia cells release lactate in response to increased energy needs. Positron emission tomography (PET) imaging studies reflecting glucose metabolism, to a significant degree, reflect glia activity. Cerebral perfusion is also significantly modulated by astroglia: on one end, astroglial extensions "sense" synaptic activity; on the other end, their distal processes, or "feet," modulate vascular tone and capillary permeability. Therefore, fMRI signals are substantially influenced by glial activity.[1,2,8]

Glial cell pathology has been reported in the subgenual anterior cingulate cortex (sgACC), dorsolateral prefrontal cortex (DLPFC), orbitofrontal cortex (OPFC), hippocampus, and the amygdala of unmedicated patients with MDD. It appears that both astroglia and oligodendroglia may be affected. Research has noted a prominent 19% reduction in oligodendroglia in the DLPFC of patients with MDD. Having in mind the crucial role that DLPFC plays in executive function and "top-down" limbic regulation, the implications of this finding are striking because it may provide a neurobiological substrate for both the emotional dysregulation and cognitive dysfunction commonly observed in MDD.[5-8]

A study using immunohistochemistry assessed microglia density in DLPFC, ACC, thalamus, and hippocampus of patients with depression. The authors suggest that significant microgliosis (i.e., increased number of microglia) in patients with depression who committed suicide relative to healthy controls might be a marker of pre-suicidal stress.[9]

In contradistinction to widespread glial abnormalities, neuronal changes appear to be subtler and more discrete in MDD. For example, some authors have noted decreased pyramidal somal size in hippocampus, ACC, DLPFC, and OPFC in postmortem studies of patients with MDD. The distribution of this cellular pathology overlaps remarkably with findings from structural and functional imaging studies. Therefore, MDD is more characterized by morphological and functional changes, rather than alterations in neuronal density.[1,5-8]

In conclusion, MDD appears to be much more a "gliopathic" rather than "neurodegenerative" disease.

REFERENCES

1. Rajkowska G, Miguel-Hidalgo JJ. Gliogenesis and glial pathology in depression. *CNS Neurol Disord Drug Targets*. 2007;6(3):219-233.
2. Pav M, Kovaru H, Fiserova A, et al. Neurobiological aspects of depressive disorder and antidepressant treatment: role of glia. *Physiol Res*. 2008;57(2):151-164.
3. Halassa MM, Fellin T, Haydon PG. The tripartite synapse: roles for gliotransmission in health and disease. *Trends Mol Med*. 2007;13(2):54-63.
4. Murai KK, Van Meyel DJ. Neuron glial communication at synapses: insights from vertebrates and invertebrates. *Neuroscientist*. 2007;13(6):657-666.
5. Rajkowska G, Miguel-Hidalgo JJ, Wei J, et al. Morphometric evidence for neuronal and glial prefrontal cell pathology in major depression. *Biol Psychiatry*. 1999;45(9):1085-1098.
6. Uranova NA, Vostrikov VM, Orlovskaya DD, Rachmanova VI. Oligodendroglial density in the prefrontal cortex in schizophrenia and mood disorders: a study from the Stanley Neuropathology Consortium. *Schizophr Res*. 2004;67(2-3):269-275.
7. Rajkowska G. Histopathology of the prefrontal cortex in major depression: what does it tell us about dysfunctional monoaminergic circuits? *Prog Brain Res*. 2000;126:397-412.
8. Maletic V, Raison CL. Neurobiology of depression, fibromyalgia and neuropathic pain. *Front Biosci*. 2009;14:5291-5338.
9. Steiner J, Bielau H, Brisch R, et al. Immunological aspects in the neurobiology of suicide: elevated microglial density in schizophrenia and depression is associated with suicide. *J Psychiatr Res*. 2008;42(2):151-157.

Hypothalamic-Pituitary-Adrenal Axis and Suicide

QUESTION: "You mentioned a link between the hypothalamic-pituitary-adrenal (HPA) axis and suicide in your *Treating the Whole Patient* presentation. Please comment further on this."

Jon W. Draud, MS, MD:

Yes, this is an interesting finding and is discussed in detail by Jokinen and Nordström.[1] Hyperactivity of the HPA axis has long been associated with patients suffering from major depressive disorder, but studies linking HPA hyperactivity and suicide are less numerous and consistent.

Jokinen and Nordström evaluated 36 inpatients under the age of 30 with (n=18) and without suicide attempt at the index episode. It has been shown that non-suppressors of the dexamethasone suppression test (DST) are more likely to commit suicide, and the results in this study seem to confirm that. The DST non-suppressor rate was 25%. It was found that DST non-suppression was associated with suicide attempt and post-dexamethasone serum cortisol at 11:00 PM, and serum cortisol levels were higher in suicide attempters compared to those who did not attempt suicide. Overall, the DST non-suppressor rate was 39% in those who attempted suicide versus 11% in those who did not attempt suicide. These results add to the established body of literature that supports a link between hyperactive HPA and suicide attempts. There were no observed gender differences in the study, and this is consistent with previous findings.

As described in a study by Claassen et al.,[2] depression with a history of suicidal behavior may be a marker for a more virulent form of depression characterized by earlier onset, more overall episodes of depressive illness, and ongoing suicidal ideation. This fits clinically with what I have observed in my practice. One point worth making is that those with early onset and frequently recurrent episodes or inadequate remission rates seem to be at a very high risk of ultimate suicidal behavior.

Clinically, this should serve as a reminder that we must be particularly diligent in assessing and monitoring this subset of patients. It also further reminds us of the critical need to strive for remission as we now know that neurobiologically, depressive illnesses seem to progress in terms of brain involvement as well as body involvement (i.e., comorbidities). Certainly, this is yet another reminder of the inextricable link between mind and body, and how one influences the other.

Finally, these data suggest that it might be wise clinically to include HPA axis measures in the overall assessment of young adults suffering with depression. Depression is a devastating illness to young and older adults, and suicide is the ultimate bad outcome of this debilitating illness. Hopefully, this example of mind-body science has given us further ideas on how to approach depression in our patients.

REFERENCES

1. Jokinen J, Nordström P. HPA axis hyperactivity and attempted suicide in young adult mood disorder inpatients. *J Affect Disord.* 2009;116(1-2):117-120.
2. Claassen CA, Trivedi MH, Rush AJ, et al. Clinical differences among depressed patients with and without a history of suicide attempts: findings from the STAR*D trial. *J Affect Disord.* 2007;97(1-3):77-84.

Neurobiology of Psychotherapy

QUESTION: **"Is therapy, such as cognitive-behavioral therapy (CBT), helpful only through psychological means, or is there a biological basis to such treatment?"**

Rakesh Jain, MD, MPH:

Psychotherapies quite clearly are nonpharmacological interventions, yet they seem to pack a powerful biological punch! This is quite a revelation for clinicians no matter what school of thought they belong to—be it purely biological or purely psychological views of depression. It is becoming very obvious that medications help not just through their effects on neurobiology, but by also affecting a patient's belief systems, which in turn exerts a powerful benefit to the individual's neurobiology. This has been demonstrated by the positive neurobiological changes that occur in patients who receive a placebo medication. In other words, there is a positive, circular relationship between positive psychological changes and positive neurobiological changes.

Psychotherapy has clearly been demonstrated to help with depression. For decades, we believed this occurred as a result of changing thought patterns. Now, this is true, but the untold story is about the neurobiology of psychotherapy. This is completely changing how we view how therapies help individuals. Let's quickly review some recent relevant studies in order to explore this issue.

Abelson and colleagues[1] recently published a study that showed that even a very brief CBT intervention was a very significant modulator of the hypothalamic-pituitary-adrenal axis, clearly revealing that a "psychological" intervention can have a strong biological impact, and do so rather quickly. This is powerful evidence that CBT is so much more than mere "let's change dysfunctional thoughts to feel better."

DeRubeis and colleagues[2] recently reviewed this issue, and found how patients dealt with negative emotions and cognitive tasks before and after they received CBT by studying blood flows in their amygdala and prefrontal cortex. Remember, not a medication study, only a psychotherapy study! The results are breathtaking—very clear and significant changes were noted pre- and post-CBT in blood flow to the brain, clearly revealing that CBT is a potent biological intervention. Interesting!

I suggest we clinicians keep our eyes on the burgeoning data emerging from the integrated psychotherapy-neurobiology literature. It appears that the time for us to adopt a true "integrative model of biology-psychology" has come, and doing so will only help us better address the needs of our mentally challenged patients.

REFERENCES
1. Abelson JL, Liberzon I, Young EA, Khan S. Cognitive modulation of endocrine stress response

to a pharmacological challenge in normal and panic disorder subjects. *Arch Gen Psychiatry*. 2005;62(6):668-675.

2. DeRubeis RJ, Siegle GJ, Hollon SD. Cognitive therapy versus medication for depression: treatment outcomes and neural mechanisms. *Nat Rev Neurosci*. 2008;9(10):788-796.

Chapter 2

**MIND-BODY CONNECTIONS OF IMMUNE
AND STRESS SYSTEMS WITH PSYCHIATRIC DISORDERS**

Depression and Inflammation: Part 1

QUESTION: "Is major depression an inflammatory disease?"

Vladimir Maletic, MS, MD:

I believe that we have strong evidence that inflammation is a relevant pathophysiological mechanism contributing to the development, severity, and persistence of major depressive disorder (MDD).[1,2,3] Is it not the same as saying that MDD is an inflammatory disease? Not, exactly. Rheumatoid arthritis and ulcerative colitis would be good examples of inflammatory disorders. Inflammation is the fundamental mechanism of etiopathogenesis in these conditions and the primary target of successful treatments. By comparison, inflammation has a significant role in etiology and propagation of malignant disorders. Yet cancers are not commonly considered as a primarily inflammatory condition, nor are the anti-inflammatory agents the mainstay of treatment.

Let us now examine the evidence linking depression and inflammation. Stress and medical illness are the principal precipitants of depression, both are associated with immune activation and elevated inflammation.[1,3] Compromised cortico-limbic regulation of mood and stress response appears to be the central feature of a depressive episode, most likely giving rise to neuropsychiatric symptoms of depression.[1,3] The brain responds to a depressed state in a manner that is very similar to a moderate "fight or flight" response: inadequate hypothalamic-pituitary-adrenal regulation, sympathetic activation combined with diminished parasympathetic tone, and, lastly, inflammation![1,3]

Evidence links elevation of proinflammatory cytokines in the context of depression to multiple somatic and psychiatric manifestations, such as change in sleep and appetite, aches, fatigue, irritability, sadness, impaired concentration and cognition, and even suicidal ideation.[1,3-6] Interferon therapy and experimentally induced inflammation are independently recognized as precipitants of depression and anxiety.[1,3] Inflammation is also a purported "missing link" explaining the synergistic impact of sleep disturbance, medical illness, and chronic stress on mood. The impact of inflammation on brain circuitry, intracellular signaling, and neuroplasticity will be discussed in another post.

REFERENCES
1. Miller AH, Maletic V, Raison CL. Inflammation and its discontents: the role of cytokines in the patho-physiology of major depression. *Biol Psychiatry*. 2009;65(9):732-741.
2. Sjögren E, Leanderson P, Kristenson M, Ernerudh J. Interleukin-6 levels in relation to psychosocial factors: studies on serum, saliva, and in vitro production by blood mononuclear cells. *Brain Behav Immun*. 2006;20(3):270-278.
3. Maletic V, Raison CL. Neurobiology of depression, fibromyalgia and neuropathic pain. *Front Biosci*. 2009;14:5291-5338.
4. Harrison NA, Brydon L, Walker C, et al. Inflammation causes mood changes through alterations in subgenual cingulated activity and mesolimbic connectivity. *Biol Psychiatry*. 2009;66(5):407-414.

5. Alesci S, Martinez PE, Kelkar S, et al. Major depression is associated with significant diurnal eleva-
    tions in plasma interleukin-6 levels, a shift of its circadian rhythm, and loss of physiological complex-
    ity in its secretion: clinical implications. *J Clin Endocrinol Metab*. 2005;90(5):2522-2530.
6. Kim YK, Na KS, Shink KH, et al. Cytokine imbalance in the pathophysiology of major depressive dis-
    order. *Prog Neuropsychopharmacol Biol Psychiatry*. 2007;31(5):1044-1053.

Depression and Inflammation: Part 2

QUESTION: "Is major depression an inflammatory disease?"

Vladimir Maletic, MS, MD:

We previously discussed the role of inflammation on the etiology and clinical presentation of depression. We will now focus our attention on an even more controversial topic: Is major depression, at least in part, a somato-psychiatric disease? In other words, do inflammatory mediators released in the course of the depressive episode directly shape neuropsychiatric symptoms of depression, and participate in functional and structural remodeling of the brain?

Let's review some available evidence. Patients suffering from depression tend to have substantially elevated peripheral levels of inflammatory cytokines (typically interleukins [IL]: IL-1, IL-6, or tumor necrosis factor-alpha).[1,2] Elevation of inflammatory mediators is a nonspecific response, commonly observed in stressful situations, even in healthy individuals.[3] What sets patients with depression apart from healthy, but "stressed-out," individuals is the lack of anti-inflammatory response (mediated by IL-10).[4] Functional imaging studies indicate that peripheral inflammatory cytokine elevation tends to be associated with activation of similar brain areas as the ones implicated in depression, pain, and stress response (amygdala, subgenual anterior cingulate [sACC], insula, and dorsolateral prefrontal cortex [DLPFC]).[2] As a matter of fact, in a group of recently vaccinated healthy individuals, elevation in peripheral inflammatory cytokines, and ensuing changes in brain activity were associated with fatigue and impaired concentration.[5] In a separate study of patients with depression, Alesci and colleagues found that elevation of plasma IL-6 directly correlated with core symptoms of depression, such as sadness, guilt, fatigue, difficulty concentrating, low self-esteem, and even suicidal ideation![6]

A growing body of pre-clinical and clinical research suggests that elevation of peripheral inflammatory cytokines may contribute to altered brain levels of serotonin and dopamine, compromised glia function, glutamate-related excitotoxicity, decline in brain-derived neurotrophic factor and other neurotrophic factors, and impaired myelination of white matter tracts connecting mood modulating prefrontal cortical and limbic areas.[1,2] Therefore, we have a good reason to believe that vicious cycle closes: peripheral inflammatory response—presumably precipitated by dysfunction of mood-regulating brain circuitry—contributes to further damage in neurotransmission, neuroplasticity, and structural integrity of critical brain areas.

REFERENCES
1. Miller AH, Maletic V, Raison CL. Inflammation and its discontents: the role of cytokines in the patho-physiology of major depression. *Biol Psychiatry*. 2009;65(9):732-741.

2. Maletic V, Raison CL. Neurobiology of depression, fibromyalgia and neuropathic pain. *Front Biosci.* 2009;14:5291-5338.

3. Raison CL, Miller AH. When not enough is too much: the role of insufficient glucocorticoid signaling in the pathophysiology of stress-related disorders. *Am J Psychiatry.* 2003;160(9):1554-1565.

4. Dhabhar FS, Burke HM, Epel ES, et al. Low serum IL-10 concentrations and loss of regulatory association between IL-6 and IL-10 in adults with major depression. *J Psychiatr Res.* 2009;43(11):962-969.

5. Harrison NA, Brydon L, Walker C, et al. Inflammation causes mood changes through alterations in subgenual cingulate activity and mesolimbic connectivity. *Biol Psychiatry.* 2009;66(5):407-414.

6. Alesci S, Martinez PE, Kelkar S, et al. Major depression is associated with significant diurnal elevations in plasma interleukin-6 levels, a shift of its circadian rhythm, and loss of physiological complexity in its secretion: clinical implications. *J Clin Endocrinol Metab.* 2005;90(5):2522-2530.

Adjunctive Anti-Inflammatory Treatment and Depression

QUESTION: **"Would use of adjunctive anti-inflammatories be useful for depression?"**

Charles Raison, MD:

The short answer to this question is maybe. I know of two randomized, placebo-controlled studies showing that the addition of the COX-2 inhibitor celecoxib significantly increased response to a noradrenergic and to a serotonergic anti-depressant.[1,2] I also know of open data suggesting that the addition of 380 mg/day of aspirin to selective serotonin reuptake inhibitors converts nonresponders to responders.[3,4] Several studies suggest that cortisone may improve depressive symptoms and be of benefit for conditions highly comorbid with depression, such as chronic fatigue syndrome,[5,6] and in patients with autoimmune disorders, several studies confirm that tumor necrosis factor (TNF)-alpha antagonists, such as infliximab or etanercept, have antidepressant properties.[7,8]

I would say that preliminary data do support the possibility that, at least in some patients, the addition of an anti-inflammatory may be useful. Remember, please, that all these agents can cause serious adverse events. This needs to be kept in the risk/benefit calculation, especially given that we are only now in the beginning of studying this issue. The data are not particularly strong yet, hence, my "maybe" answer.

REFERENCES
1. Akhondzadeh S, Jafari S, Raisi F, et al. Clinical trial of adjunctive celecoxib treatment in patients with major depression: a double blind and placebo controlled trial. *Depress Anxiety*. 2009;26(7):607-611.
2. Muller N, Schwarz MJ, Dehning S, et al. The cyclooxygenase-2 inhibitor celecoxib has therapeutic effects in major depression: results of a double-blind, randomized, placebo controlled, add-on pilot study to reboxetine. *Mol Psychiatry*. 2006;11(7):680-684.
3. Mendlewicz J, Kriwin P, Oswald P, Souery D, et al. Shortened onset of action of antidepressants in major depression using acetylsalicylic acid augmentation: a pilot open-label study. *Int Clin Psychopharmacol*. 2006;21(4):227-231.
4. Brunello N, Alboni S, Capone G, et al. Acetylsalicylic acid accelerates the antidepressant effect of fluoxetine in the chronic escape deficit model of depression. *Int Clin Psychopharmacol*. 2006;21(4):219-225.
5. Goodwin GM, Muir WJ, Seckl JR, et al. The effects of cortisol infusion upon hormone secretion from the anterior pituitary and subjective mood in depressive illness and in controls. *J Affect Disord*. 1992;26(2):73-83.
6. McKenzie R, O'Fallon A, Dale J, et al. Low-dose hydrocortisone for treatment of chronic fatigue syndrome: a randomized controlled trial. *JAMA*. 1998;280(12):1061-1066.
7. Persoons P, Vermeire S, Demyttenaere K, et al. The impact of major depressive disorder on the short- and long-term outcome of Crohn's disease treatment with infliximab. *Aliment Pharmacol Ther*. 2005;22(2):101-110.
8. Tyring S, Gottlieb A, Papp K, et al. Etanercept and clinical outcomes, fatigue, and depression in psoriasis: double-blind placebo-controlled randomised phase III trial. *Lancet*. 2006;367(9504):29-35.

Treating Depression with Anti-Inflammatory Agents

QUESTION: "Would treating the actual cascade of immune response also treat depression, i.e., target cytokines?"

Charles Raison, MD:

This is a great question with a simple answer, which is that we don't know the answer, at least not yet. You've come to the right place because—along with Andrew H. Miller, MD—I am principal investigator for a government grant that has allowed us to examine whether a very potent anti-inflammatory agent called infliximab is an effective antidepressant in people who are medically healthy but have treatment-resistant depression. This week, Dr. Miller and I opened a bottle of champagne surreptitiously in our offices to celebrate the fact that we had enrolled our 60th and final participant in the study. This participant will complete the study in three months, after which we will very quickly know whether directly blocking the proinflammatory cytokine tumor necrosis factor (TNF)-alpha (which is the mechanism of action for infliximab) treats depression.

If infliximab treats depression, that will provide a simple and compelling answer to your question. If it doesn't work that doesn't necessarily mean that blocking cytokines is a failed strategy; however, because infliximab is too large a molecule to get into the brain, it is possible that blockade of cytokine activity within the central nervous system is required for antidepressant efficacy. Of course, if infliximab does work for depression, this makes a strong argument for the fact that bodily inflammation is important in and of itself in modulating brain states.

To our knowledge, no other studies have been conducted that directly examine whether cytokine antagonists treat depression in people who are medically healthy. However, several studies suggest that these agents have antidepressant properties in people with diseases known to be associated with increased inflammation. For example, in a large study of patients with psoriasis, Tyring et al. found that the TNF-alpha antagonist etanercept was more effective than placebo in lowering depression scores.[1] Moreover, the changes in depression were not associated with improvements in the underlying medical condition, suggesting direct anti-inflammatory activity for the cytokine blocker. Similarly, antidepressant efficacy has been observed for infliximab in patients with Crohn's disease.[2]

Although not cytokine blockers per se, agents that inhibit cyclooxygenase (COX) have potent anti-inflammatory properties by reducing the production of prostaglandins that are key components of the inflammatory cascade. Two randomized, double-blind studies found that the addition of the COX-2 inhibitor celecoxib to a selective serotonin reuptake inhibitor (SSRI) led to a greater reduction in depressive symptoms than the addition of a placebo.[3,4] Using a similar design, celecoxib was also found to be an effective augmenting strategy for reducing symptoms in bipolar patients in a depressed or mixed state.[5]

For years, whenever I lectured about depression being associated with increased inflammation, someone would raise a hand and sagely challenge me by asking, "Doesn't this mean that aspirin should help depression?" I always had to admit yes without realizing that, by 2006, an open trial had shown that the addition of aspirin to medically healthy patients with major depression who had failed four weeks of SSRI treatment led to a rapid and profound improvement in just over half the sample.[6]

In summary, you've asked your very cogent question about six months to a year too soon. By that time, we'll know how promising the direct blockade of proinflammatory cytokines is for treating major depression. In addition, big studies are afoot in Europe that are examining whether COX-2 inhibitors really work to augment antidepressants, and whether they might be antidepressants in and of themselves. Stay tuned.

REFERENCES

1. Tyring S, Gottlieb A, Papp K, et al. Etanercept and clinical outcomes, fatigue, and depression in psoriasis: double-blind placebo-controlled randomised phase III trial. *Lancet*. 2006;367(9504):29-35.

2. Persoons P, Vermeire S, Demyttenaere K, et al. The impact of major depressive disorder on the short- and long-term outcome of Crohn's disease treatment with infliximab. *Aliment Pharmacol Ther*. 2005;22(2):101-110.

3. Akhondzadeh S, Jafari S, Raisi F, et al. Clinical trial of adjunctive celecoxib treatment in patients with major depression: a double blind and placebo controlled trial. *Depress Anxiety*. 2009;26(7):607-611.

4. Muller N, Schwarz MJ, Dehning S, et al. The cyclooxygenase-2 inhibitor celecoxib has therapeutic effects in major depression: results of a double-blind, randomized, placebo controlled, add-on pilot study to reboxetine. *Mol Psychiatry*. 2006;11(7):680-684.

5. Nery FG, Monkul ES, Hatch JP, et al. Celecoxib as an adjunct in the treatment of depressive or mixed episodes of bipolar disorder: a double-blind, randomized, placebo-controlled study. *Hum Psychopharmacol*. 2008;23(2):87-94.

6. Mendlewicz J, Kriwin P, Oswald P, Souery D, Alboni S, Brunello N. Shortened onset of action of antidepressants in major depression using acetylsalicylic acid augmentation: a pilot open-label study. *Int Clin Psychopharmacol*. 2006;21(4):227-231.

Interferon-Induced Mania

QUESTION: "Have you seen interferon precipitate mania in a patient?"

Charles Raison, MD:

I most definitely have. My experience in this regard is consistent with many case reports describing people who were psychiatrically normal prior to commencing therapy with the cytokine interferon (IFN)-alpha for either cancer or chronic hepatitis C virus infection.[1-4] Our best data suggest that between 20% to 50% of people will meet criteria for major depression at some point during treatment with IFN-alpha,[4] and 1% to 2% will develop classic euphoric manias.[2] Many more people will develop a mixture of symptoms that defy easy categorization, but that includes a mixture of irritability, racing thoughts, anxiety, fatigue, and anhedonia. The best study of this phenomenon was done by a group in Bordeaux, France. By applying strict *Diagnostic and Statistical Manual of Mental Disorders-IV* (*DSM-IV*) criteria, they determined that most people who qualified for a mood disorder diagnosis were best classified depressive mixed states.[2]

We know from many studies that IFN-alpha tends to magnify people's baseline condition. For example, the most replicated risk factor for developing clinical depression during treatment is having any level of depressive and/or anxiety symptoms prior to starting.[4,5] We suspect the same thing is true for treatment-emergent mania; that is, that people with premorbid bipolar disorder are more likely to have them during IFN-alpha treatment, but this has never been definitively established. Similarly, no one has ever conducted a rigorous study of how to best treat IFN-alpha-induced manias, but lots of clinical experience suggests that these episodes respond to mood stabilizers/antipsychotics as do idiopathic manias. On the other hand, we have a fair amount of data for how to treat depression during IFN-alpha. Studies show that the incidence of IFN-alpha depression can be reduced by pretreatment with an antidepressant,[6-8] but work by our group shows that antidepressant pretreatment only seems to benefit individuals with at least mild depression or anxiety symptoms prior to treatment.[6] Studies also suggest that antidepressants are effective in treating mood disorder symptoms once they have developed during IFN-alpha treatment.[9,10]

For the clinician, the high burden of psychiatric side effects that accompany IFN-alpha are a primary treatment challenge. For those of us who are also researchers, however, IFN-alpha has provided a truly unique opportunity to understand how the immune system contributes to the development of mood disorders. Because it is increasingly clear that psychological stress activates inflammation,[11,12] as does sickness, findings from IFN-alpha really extend out—we suspect—to mood disorders in general, even in medically healthy individuals. What we and other research groups have found is that people who develop depression in response to IFN-alpha develop many of the same physiological changes that have been reported for mood disorders in general, including glucocorticoid resistance, flattening of the diurnal cortisol rhythm, sleep disruption and reduced slow wave sleep, impairments in the metabolism of tryptophan (leading to serotonergic changes), and the generation of excitotoxic/neurotoxic chemicals in the central nervous system.[13-16]

Not enough people develop pure manias during IFN-alpha treatment for it to be studied in the same way that depression has been studied. However, I suspect that many of the same physiological changes seen during IFN-alpha depression would also be observed during IFN-alpha-induced mania. I say this because data increasingly suggest that "regular" manias look very similar to depression in many ways. Why should IFN-alpha-induced mania be any different?

Let me close with a final practical point about manias associated with IFN-alpha. Patients seem to be at risk not only during treatment itself, but also in the weeks to months following treatment. I've seen this with my own eyes. We had a research participant who developed such severe depression we had to discontinue her from the study. In defiance of our advice, she did not immediately go to a clinician to start an antidepressant. Two weeks after stopping the IFN-alpha, she began to develop racing thoughts, mild grandiosity, increased goal directed activity, and decreased need for sleep.

Fortunately, although the severity of her symptoms probably crossed the line into full mania, she did not get into trouble and the episode spontaneously resolved over the course of a week or two. The take-home point here is that if you treat people undergoing therapy with IFN-alpha you really need to keep a close eye on them after they finish therapy, and not just while they are in its throes.

REFERENCES

1. Adams F, Fernandez F, Mavligit G. Interferon-induced organic mental disorders associated with unsuspected pre-existing neurologic abnormalities. *J Neurooncol*. 1988;6(4):355-359.
2. Constant A, Castera L, Dantzer R, et al. Mood alterations during interferon-alfa therapy in patients with chronic hepatitis C: evidence for an overlap between manic/hypomanic and depressive symptoms. *J Clin Psychiatry*. 2005;66(8):1050-1057.
3. Greenberg DB, Jonasch E, Gadd MA, et al. Adjuvant therapy of melanoma with interferon-alpha-2b is associated with mania and bipolar syndromes. *Cancer*. 2000;89(2):356-362.
4. Raison CL, Demetrashvili M, Capuron L, Miller AH. Neuropsychiatric adverse effects of interferon-alpha: recognition and management. *CNS Drugs*. 2005;19(2):105-123.
5. Raison CL, Borisov AS, Broadwell SD, et al. Depression during pegylated interferon-alpha plus ribavirin therapy: prevalence and prediction. *J Clin Psychiatry*. 2005;66(1):41-48.
6. Raison CL, Woolwine BJ, Demetrashvili MF, et al. Paroxetine for prevention of depressive symptoms induced by interferon-alpha and ribavirin for hepatitis C. *Aliment Pharmacol Ther*. 2007;25(10):1163-1174.
7. Musselman DL, Lawson DH, Gumnick JF, et al. Paroxetine for the prevention of depression induced by high-dose interferon alfa. *N Engl J Med*. 2001;344(13):961-966.
8. Kraus MR, Schafer A, Al-Taie O, Scheurlen M. Prophylactic SSRI during interferon alpha re-therapy in patients with chronic hepatitis C and a history of interferon-induced depression. *J Viral Hepat*. 2005;12(1):96-100.
9. Kraus MR, Schafer A, Schottker K, et al. Therapy of interferon-induced depression in chronic hepatitis C with citalopram: a randomised, double-blind, placebo-controlled study. *Gut*. 2008;57(4):531-536.

10. Loftis JM, Hauser P. The phenomenology and treatment of interferon-induced depression. *J Affect Disord*. 2004;82(2):175-190.
11. Pace TW, Mletzko TC, Alagbe O, et al. Increased stress-induced inflammatory responses in male patients with major depression and increased early life stress. *Am J Psychiatry*. 2006;163(9):1630-1633.
12. Steptoe A, Hamer M, Chida Y. The effect of acute psychological stress on circulating inflammatory factors in humans: a review and meta-analysis. *Brain Behav Immun*. 2007;21(7):901-912.
13. Raison CL, Rye DB, Woolwine BJ, et al. Chronic interferon-alpha administration disrupts sleep continuity and depth in patients with hepatitis C: association with fatigue, motor slowing, and increased evening cortisol. *Biol Psychiatry*. 2010;68(10):942-949.
14. Raison CL, Dantzer R, Kelley KW, et al. CSF concentrations of brain tryptophan and kynurenines during immune stimulation with IFN-alpha: relationship to CNS immune responses and depression. *Mol Psychiatry*. 2010;15(4):393-403.
15. Raison CL, Borisov AS, Woolwine BJ, et al. Interferon-alpha effects on diurnal hypothalamic-pituitary-adrenal axis activity: relationship with proinflammatory cytokines and behavior. *Mol Psychiatry*. 2010;15(5):535-547.
16. Raison CL, Borisov AS, Majer M, et al. Activation of central nervous system inflammatory pathways by interferon-alpha: relationship to monoamines and depression. *Biol Psychiatry*. 2009;65(4):296-303.

Hepatitis C Virus and Depression

QUESTION: **"By treating people with antidepressants who are taking interferon for hepatitis are we interfering with halting the virus?"**

Charles Raison, MD:

This is a great question that shows a good grasp of immunology. We give people with hepatitis C virus (HCV) infection interferon (IFN)-alpha because, as a pro-inflammatory cytokine, IFN-alpha activates the immune system to better rid the body of the virus. Many studies suggest that antidepressants reduce inflammatory signaling. If they do this, maybe they interfere with the action of IFN-alpha, which would lead to a terrible irony. People would feel better on an antidepressant but at the price of going through the miseries of IFN-alpha for nothing, or at least a better chance of a bad outcome.

The answer is—unfortunately—that no one knows.[1] Our group was involved in planning what would have been a huge study testing this issue. This study was actually designed to show the opposite—that antidepressant pretreatment would improve viral outcomes because people would be more likely to be able to stay on IFN-alpha as a result of improved side-effect burden. We spent the better part of a year working on it, but it was killed at the FDA, and with that, the opportunity to perform a really rigorous examination probably vanished for all time.

What do we know? Well, a corollary of antidepressants interfering with viral response to IFN-alpha would be that depression during IFN-alpha treatment should be a good thing, because it reflects increased inflammation that is also helping clear the virus. So you would predict that the more depressed people get during treatment, the more likely they will be to clear HCV. Here is what we know: Loftis and colleagues[2] reported that patients who developed major depression during IFN-alpha/ribavirin therapy were more likely to achieve a sustained viral response. But here's the wrinkle: patients who developed major depression were also the only ones started on an antidepressant—and as a group they had significant and immediate reductions in their depression scores. Maybe it was the addition of an antidepressant that improved viral response? In contradistinction to the Loftis et al. findings, our group reported a strong association between increases in depressive symptoms during IFN-alpha/ribavirin treatment and reduced rates of viral clearance.[3] A similar result was found by Maddock et al.[4] who observed an association between increased fatigue scores and decreased viral clearance (with fatigue being a prominent depressive symptom).

Although these findings seem contradictory, there appears upon closer inspection to be an underlying pattern. When depression is measured as a maximal score attained during treatment, the correlation between depression and viral clearance is weaker than when depression is measured as amount of change from baseline.

When considered this way, there seems to be a consistent signal that increases in depression, which is bad for viral clearance. I think that amount of change from baseline is a more relevant measure at any rate, because how high a depression score people achieve during treatment is very much related to how high a score they have before they start treatment.[5] While measuring severity has clear clinical implications important for managing people during IFN-alpha treatment, the amount of increase in depression is almost certainly more related to direct cytokine effects that are also linked to viral clearance.

I have a bias, as you can tell. I find it very hard to believe that depression can be good for much of anything. Can anyone think of any medical condition in which developing depression is a good thing for health outcomes? Quite the contrary, in every condition I know of, developing depression significantly worsens morbidity and frequently increases mortality, too. It turns out that although inflammation evolved to fight pathogens, it can also cause at least as much trouble as benefit when it comes to disease outcomes, so one shouldn't just expect that more inflammation is a good thing when it comes to clearing an infection like HCV. In fact, many studies suggest that people who have increased inflammatory markers prior to commencing IFN-alpha treatment don't do as well. Similarly, overly robust inflammatory responses to IFN-alpha (which we and others have shown are associated with increased depression)[6,7] predict <u>NOT</u> clearing virus. The reason for this isn't totally clear, but likely has to do with the fact that inflammatory processes when excessive or prolonged can actually impair virus specific T cell activity. This line of reasoning has led to an interesting series of studies now in progress that involve giving cytokine antagonists to patients receiving IFN-alpha for HCV to improve their viral outcomes.

So all in all, I think current data do not strongly suggest that using antidepressants during IFN-alpha therapy will negatively impact viral outcomes, but again let me stress that we do not have adequate data to make firm conclusions. Of course, the use of antidepressants during IFN-alpha treatment is widespread, so let me close by commenting on this in practical terms. Many clinicians routinely start an antidepressant in everyone who is about to undergo IFN-alpha treatment. Let me suggest that currently available data do not necessarily support this practice. I know of only two randomized, double-blind studies testing this practice in patients with HCV. One study was negative,[8] and the other showed that while antidepressant pretreatment worked, it only worked in patients who had mild anxiety and depression prior to starting IFN-alpha.[9] This suggests that vulnerable patients (i.e., those with pre-existing psychiatric issues) probably benefit from antidepressant pretreatment, whereas people without such struggles are probably better served by starting IFN-alpha and then adding an antidepressant if depression emerges. A well-done recent study from Europe demonstrates the effectiveness of this type of rescue strategy.[10] Finally, antidepressants are not a cure all for the problems induced by IFN-alpha. They are more effective for emotional symptoms (i.e., depressed mood, anxiety) than they are for bothersome somatic symptoms frequently induced by IFN-alpha, including fatigue, sleep disturbance, and loss of appetite.[11] Sadly, no one has ever adequately studied how to best address these symptoms, which—by the way—also auger a bad outcome in "regular old" depression, as attested to by a recent review of the literature.[12]

REFERENCES

1. Robaeys G, Wichers MC, De Bie J, et al. Does antidepressant medication in patients with hepatitis C undergoing interferon alpha treatment reduce therapeutic efficacy? *Gut.* 2009;58(1):145; author reply 145-146.
2. Loftis JM, Socherman RE, Howell CD, et al. Association of interferon-alpha-induced depression and improved treatment repsonse in patients with hepatitis C. *Neurosci Lett.* 2004;365(2):87-91.
3. Raison CL, Broadwell SD, Borisov AS, et al. Depressive symptoms and viral clearance in patients receiving interferon-alpha and ribavirin for hepatitis C. *Brain Behav and Immun.* 2005;19(1):23-27.
4. Maddock C, Landau S, Barry K, et al. Psychopathological symptoms during interferon-alpha and ribavirin treatment: effects on virologic response. *Mol Psychiatry.* 2005;10(4):332-333.
5. Raison CL, Borisov AS, Broadwell SD, et al. Depression during pegylated interferon-alpha plus ribavirin therapy: prevalence and prediction. *J Clin Psychiatry.* 2005;66(1):41-48.
6. Raison CL, Borisov AS, Woolwine BJ, et al. Interferon-alpha effects on diurnal hypothalamic-pituitary-adrenal axis activity: relationship with proinflammatory cytokines and behavior. *Mol Psychiatry.* Jun 3 2008.
7. Prather AA, Rabinovitz M, Pollock BG, Lotrich FE. Cytokine-induced depression during IFN-alpha treatment: the role of IL-6 and sleep quality. *Brain Behav Immun.* 2009;23(8):1109-1116.
8. Morasco BJ, Rifai MA, Loftis JM, et al. A randomized trial of paroxetine to prevent interferon-alpha-induced depression in patients with hepatitis C. *J Affect Disord.* 2007;103(1-3):83-90.
9. Raison CL, Woolwine BJ, Demetrashvili MF, et al. Paroxetine for prevention of depressive symptoms induced by interferon-alpha and ribavirin for hepatitis C. *Aliment Pharmacol Ther.* 2007;25(10):1163-1174.
10. Kraus MR, Schafer A, Schottker K, et al. Therapy of interferon-induced depression in chronic hepatitis C with citalopram: a randomised, double-blind, placebo-controlled study. *Gut.* 2008;57(4):531-536.
11. Capuron L, Gumnick JF, Musselman DL, et al. Neurobehavioral effects of interferon-alpha in cancer patients: phenomenology and paroxetine responsiveness of symptom dimensions. *Neuropsychopharmacology.* 2002;26(5):643-652.
12. Huijbregts KML, van der Feltz-Cornelis CM, van Marwijk HWJ, et al. Negative association of concomitant physical symptoms with the course of major depressive disorder: a systematic review. *J Psychosom Res.* 2010;[Epub ahead of print].

Antidepressant Pretreatment and Chemotherapy

QUESTION: "In cancer treatment, should patients undergoing chemotherapy be premedicated with anti-anxiety medications or antidepressants (with or without symptoms of anxiety or depression) to help them feel more responsive to chemotherapy by reducing inflammation in the body? Discuss the pros and cons of this idea."

Charles Raison, MD:

This question shows great understandings of the implications of the role of inflammatory pathways in major depression. The gist of the issue comes down to this: If cancer and its treatment induce inflammation, and inflammation promotes depression, then pretreating cancer patients prior to chemotherapy initiation might block negative mood effects of the treatment. On the other hand, if inflammation is required to kill the cancer, then perhaps such a strategy might come at too high a cost. Who cares about feeling better if this impairs the reason for going to all the trouble in the first place?

Let's address the first issue, and then the second. In fact, a number of studies suggest that antidepressant pretreatment can ameliorate the development of depression, not just in response to cancer chemotherapy but to other medical interventions that are also associated with inflammation. In terms of chemotherapy, the classic study was done by Andy Miller and Dominique Musselman at Emory just before I joined the Mind-Body group there. Based on studies in animals showing that antidepressants can prevent sickness behavior,[1] Andy and Dominique hypothesized that antidepressant pretreatment might also reduce the high rate of depression that occurs during treatment with the cytokine interferon (IFN)-alpha. IFN-alpha forms a mainstay of treatment for several neoplasms—including malignant melanoma and renal cell carcinoma—and for chronic hepatitis C virus (HCV) infection.[2] It doesn't work very well for cancer, but has high rates of success for HCV. To test their theory, 40 participants with non-metastatic malignant melanoma, without significant depressive or anxiety symptoms, were randomized to receive either paroxetine or placebo, commencing two weeks before IFN-alpha initiation and continuing throughout treatment. Consistent with prior reports, almost 50% of patients receiving IFN-alpha plus placebo developed symptomatic criteria for major depression over the first three months of treatment, compared to only 11% in the group that received paroxetine.[3] This antidepressant response had practical consequences. 35% of the patients receiving IFN-alpha plus placebo elected to discontinue the IFN-alpha due to severe depressive symptoms, whereas only 5% discontinued for similar reasons in the paroxetine-treated group.

As far as I know this is the only randomized, double-blind study of antidepressant prophylaxis initiated prior to cancer chemotherapy. But similar results were observed in a far larger study of cancer patients conducted by Morrow and colleagues. These investigators hypothesized that selective serotonin reuptake inhibitors (SSRI) would improve chemotherapy-induced fatigue. To test this theory, they randomized 549 participants who had developed fatigue after an initial course of chemotherapy to either paroxetine or placebo and then followed these participants through several more rounds of chemotherapy. Paroxetine showed no benefit for fatigue, but significantly reduced chemotherapy-associated depressive symptoms.[4] Interestingly, when Lucile Capuron from our group went back and looked more closely at data on paroxetine pretreatment for IFN-alpha treatment of malignant melanoma, she found a similar result. The SSRI had completely blocked the development of sad mood, anxiety, and irritability, but had been no better than placebo in reducing fatigue, sleep, or appetite.[5] These data suggest that SSRIs are more effective in reducing the emotional symptoms of depression than they are in reducing somatic symptoms. A similar pattern has been observed in medically healthy patients with depression.[6] Whether other classes of antidepressants would be more effective choices for chemotherapy prophylaxis has never been rigorously examined.

Several studies have extended the work on antidepressant pretreatment prior to IFN-alpha therapy by examining patients receiving the cytokine for HCV. In general, these studies suggest that—as with malignant melanoma—SSRIs initiated prior to IFN-alpha can reduce the development of depression.[7] Not all studies find this.[8] If one looks closely at the literature, however, a consistent pattern emerges. As our group showed several years ago, people without premorbid risk factors are not likely to develop clinically relevant depressive symptoms in response to the lower doses of IFN-alpha used to treat HCV and do not benefit much from antidepressant pretreatment.[9] On the other hand, even mildly increased depression or anxiety prior to treatment significantly increases the risk of IFN-alpha-induced depression. And people who are even a little bit down or anxious prior to IFN-alpha therapy do much better in terms of behavioral side effects if they receive antidepressant pretreatment.[9]

These findings remind me of a verse from the Bible: "To those who have more will be given." This aptly describes how to think about who is at risk for developing depression in response to any depressogenic challenge, not just cytokine therapy. People with a past history of depression and/or with current subsyndromal depressive and anxiety symptoms are primed to run into trouble in the face of environmental adversity, be it immunological or psychological. Our group and others have also identified a number of physiological risks for developing depression. For example, we have shown that the more of the stress hormone cortisol the body makes in response to a first dose of IFN-alpha, the more likely a person is to be depressed after two months of IFN-alpha treatment for malignant melanoma.[10] We and others have observed that increased levels of proinflammatory cytokines prior to treatment seem to confer a similar risk for developing depression under the strain of IFN-alpha-induced chronic inflammatory activation.[11]

Although IFN-alpha is the best studied chemotherapeutic agent in terms of antidepressant prophylaxis, similar results have been shown in several other oncological treatment settings. For example, pretreatment with fluoxetine prior to adjuvant chemotherapy for breast cancer was found to reduce depressive symptoms, improve quality of life, and lead to higher chemotherapy completion rates over a six month period.[12] Similarly, pretreatment with citalopram prior to chemotherapy for head and neck cancer reduced depressive symptoms and reduced deterioration in quality of life.[13]

That is a quick summary of the literature on antidepressant pretreatment for cancer chemotherapy. Now to the second issue, which is the question of whether antidepressants might impede therapeutic response by lowering inflammation. Studies have gone back and forth on whether antidepressant use in general is a risk factor for cancer development or progression, and my take on this literature is that the answer is most likely no. In fact, recent research suggests that SSRIs might actually have tumor fighting potential, especially in gastrointestinal cancers.[14] Perhaps these complications are to be expected because a complex relationship exists between inflammation and cancer. On the one hand, inflammatory processes are an essential component in immune-based defense against oncogenesis. But on the other hand, data increasingly implicate the body's inflammatory activity in multiple aspects of cancer development and spread. Even mild elevations in inflammatory markers have been shown in prospective studies to increase the risk for cancer development.[15] Inflammation has been repeatedly implicated in metastatic processes.[16] Finally, inflammation contributes significantly to the development of resistance to chemotherapy.[17] Not surprisingly, given all this, novel anti-inflammatory strategies are at the forefront of novel chemotherapeutic agent development.[18]

How would I summarize all this? I think data support the use of antidepressant prophylaxis for vulnerable patients being exposed to any proinflammatory medical situation. Many lines of evidence suggest that most of us have more inflammation than we need to optimally fight modern wear-and-tear disorders such as cancer or cardiovascular disease, so I think it is likely that—other things being equal—antidepressants are more likely to help, or be neutral, in regard to medical outcomes than to harm patients. Data for antidepressant prophylaxis are best for IFN-alpha, but I would consider this strategy in the face of any serious or long-term medical/surgical intervention. Vulnerable individuals include those with a past history of depression and/or with anxiety or depressive symptoms prior to the immune challenge.

REFERENCES

1. Dantzer R, O'Connor JC, Freund GG, et al. From inflammation to sickness and depression: when the immune system subjugates the brain. *Nat Rev Neurosci*. 2008;9(1):46-56.
2. Raison CL, Demetrashvili M, Capuron L, Miller AH. Neuropsychiatric adverse effects of interferon-alpha: recognition and management. *CNS Drugs*. 2005;19(2):105-123.
3. Musselman DL, Lawson DH, Gumnick JF, et al. Paroxetine for the prevention of depression induced by high-dose interferon alfa. *N Engl J Med*. 2001;344(13):961-966.

4. Morrow GR, Hickok JT, Roscoe JA, et al. Differential effects of paroxetine on fatigue and depression: a randomized, double-blind trial from the University of Rochester Cancer Center Community Clinical Oncology Program. *J Clin Oncol.* 2003;21(24):4635-4641.

5. Capuron L, Gumnick JF, Musselman DL, et al. Neurobehavioral effects of interferon-alpha in cancer patients: phenomenology and paroxetine responsiveness of symptom dimensions. *Neuropsychopharmacology.* 2002;26(5):643-652.

6. Greco T, Eckert G, Kroenke K. The outcome of physical symptoms with treatment of depression. *J Gen Intern Med.* 2004;19(8):813-818.

7. Galvao-de Almeida A, Guindalini C, Batista-Neves S, et al. Can antidepressants prevent interferon-alpha-induced depression? A review of the literature. *Gen Hosp Psychiatry.* 2010;32(4):401-405.

8. Morasco BJ, Rifai MA, Loftis JM, et al. A randomized trial of paroxetine to prevent interferon-alpha-induced depression in patients with hepatitis C. *J Affect Disord.* 2007;103(1-3):83-90.

9. Raison CL, Woolwine BJ, Demetrashvili MF, et al. Paroxetine for prevention of depressive symptoms induced by interferon-alpha and ribavirin for hepatitis C. *Aliment Pharm Ther.* 2007;25(10):1163-1174.

10. Capuron L, Raison CL, Musselman DL, et al. Association of exaggerated HPA axis response to the initial injection of interferon-alpha with development of depression during interferon-alpha therapy. *Am J Psychiatry.* 2003;160(7):1342-1345.

11. Lotrich FE. Major depression during interferon-alpha treatment: vulnerability and prevention. *Dialogues Clin Neurosci.* 2009;11(4):417-425.

12. Navari RM, Brenner MC, Wilson MN. Treatment of depressive symptoms in patients with early stage breast cancer undergoing adjuvant therapy. *Breast Cancer Res Treat.* 2008;112(1):197-201.

13. Lydiatt WM, Denman D, McNeilly DP, et al. A randomized, placebo-controlled trial of citalopram for the prevention of major depression during treatment for head and neck cancer. *Arch Otolaryngol Head Neck Surg.* 2008;134(5):528-535.

14. Argov M, Kashi R, Peer D, Margalit R. Treatment of resistant human colon cancer xenografts by a fluoxetine-doxorubicin combination enhances therapeutic responses comparable to an aggressive bevacizumab regimen. *Cancer Lett.* 2009;274(1):118-125.

15. Trompet S, de Craen AJ, Mooijaart S, et al. High innate production capacity of proinflammatory cytokines increases risk for death from cancer: results of the PROSPER Study. *Clin Cancer Res.* 2009;15(24):7744-7748.

16. Hiratsuka S, Watanabe A, Aburatani H, Maru Y. Tumour-mediated upregulation of chemoattractants and recruitment of myeloid cells predetermines lung metastasis. *Nat Cell Biol.* 2006;8(12):1369-1375.

17. Izzo JG, Correa AM, Wu TT, et al. Pretherapy nuclear factor-kappaB status, chemoradiation resistance, and metastatic progression in esophageal carcinoma. *Mol Cancer Ther.* 2006;5(11):2844-2850.

18. Anand P, Thomas SG, Kunnumakkara AB, et al. Biological activities of curcumin and its analogues (Congeners) made by man and Mother Nature. *Biochem Pharmacol.* 2008;76(11):1590-1611.

Cardiovascular Disease and Depression

QUESTION: "Could you please comment on the relationship between depression and cardiovascular disease?"

Jon W. Draud, MS, MD:

This is an excellent question that underscores the mind-body connection. The connection between depression and cardiovascular illness is quite robust and there is a wealth of literature to support it. Essentially, due to a hyperactive hypothalamic-pituitary-adrenal axis we believe that there are alterations in the periphery of cytokine levels, cortisol levels, and catecholaminergic tone. This primes the heart and other organ systems for numerous diseases.

I would like to examine several studies to illustrate the point further. First, Whang and colleagues[1] looked at over 63,000 patients and illustrated a correlation between depression status and sudden cardiac death, fatal coronary disease, and non-fatal myocardial infarction (MI).

There is also an impressive paper by Patten and colleagues[2] that examined the cumulative incidence of high blood pressure in patients with major depression versus without major depression. The study evaluated over 12,000 patients during 10 years of follow up. After age adjustment, there was a 60% increased risk of developing high blood pressure in patients with major depression (hazard ratio = 1.6).

Benton and colleagues[3] published an impressive paper in *Annals of Clinical Psychiatry* wherein they demonstrated that coronary heart disease influenced survival curves in patients with depression versus patients without depression.

Looking further, Lespérance and colleagues[4] examined post-MI patients in a hospital who were screened for depression with the Beck Depression Inventory (BDI). The initial depression score was shown to correlate with long-term survival post-MI.

A British study by Surtees and colleagues[5] demonstrated an increased risk for ischemic heart disease in patients with major depression wherein almost 20,000 patients were studied. The findings were quite interesting. Patients who were currently depressed had the highest risk for ischemic heart disease, and those who were depressed within the past 12 months also had elevated risk, but those who had suffered previously but had been in remission for 12 months or greater had no elevated risk from baseline. This challenges us as clinicians to diagnose and treat depression aggressively.

Whereas the data demonstrating this association between depression and cardiovascular illness is so numerous that we could go on for hours, I will present for your consideration one last study. Frasure-Smith and colleagues[6] evaluated depressive symptoms as measured by BDI scores, as well as C-reactive protein levels. These results again demonstrated that both depression levels, as well as inflammatory cytokine levels, were negatively associated with cardiac survival in a two-year study of 741 patients with acute coronary syndrome.

It is hoped that this discussion will further stimulate us as clinicians to appreciate the strong association between depression and cardiovascular illnesses. We, as clinicians, should be diligent in screening patients for depression when they present wtih cardiovascular disease and vice versa.

REFERENCES

1. Whang W, Kubzansky LD, Kawachi I, et al. Depression and risk of sudden cardiac death and coronary heart disease in women: results from the Nurses' Health Study. *J Am Coll Cardiol.* 2009;53(11):950-958.

2. Patten SB, Williams JV, Lavorato DH, et al. Major depression as a risk factor for high blood pressure: epidemiologic evidence from a national longitudinal study. *Psychosom Med.* 2009;71(3):273-279.

3. Benton T, Staab J, Evans DL. Medical co-morbidity in depressive disorders. *Ann Clin Psychiatry.* 2007;19(4):289-303.

4. Lespérance F, Frasure-Smith N, Talajic M, Bourassa MG. Five-year risk of cardiac mortality in relation to initial severity and one-year changes in depression after myocardial infaction. *Circulation.* 2002;105(9):1049-1053.

5. Surtees PG, Wainwright NW, Luben RN, et al. Depression and ischemic heart disease mortality: evidence from the EPIC-Norfolk United Kingdom prospective cohort study. *Am J Psychiatry.* 2008;165(4):515-523.

6. Frasure-Smith N, Lespérance F, Irwin MR, et al. Depression, C-reactive protein and two-year major adverse cardiac events in men after acute coronary syndromes. *Biol Psychiatry.* 2007;62(4):302-308.

Biological Test for Depression

QUESTION: "Why doesn't psychiatry use the serial levels of brain-derived neurotrophic factor (BDNF) and the cytokines as strong markers for the diagnosis of depression and in the assessment of the effectiveness of treatment as it is done for cardiac enzymes in the diagnosis of myocardial infarction (MI)?"

Charles Raison, MD:

I am glad you asked this question, because it actually touches upon what I consider to be the central conceptual shift we need to make in our understanding of psychiatric disease, in general, and major depression, in particular. As a start to answering this, let's ask another question: Why would we want to get serial levels of bodily chemicals, such as BDNF or cytokines? If you think about it for awhile, I suspect you will agree that the only reason to go through all the trouble would be because measuring the chemicals would tell you something you can't "see with the naked eye." What sort of questions would be important for any blood test for depression to answer? In general, three things: 1) Does the patient have a certain illness; 2) Is there a specific treatment that would be best suited to this particular patient; and 3) What is this patient's prognosis—what can she or he expect from the disease?

Let's start with the first question. The hope that someday we'll have a blood test for depression is one of the longest-standing fantasies of our field. I want to suggest that it is profoundly misguided, because it really misunderstands the type of entity depression is. Can you cut depression out of a person like a tumor and show it to me? Of course not. It is a probabilistic syndrome. It is a chronic tendency for a person to experience dark emotions, loss of interest, and any of a number of related cognitive and neurovegetative symptoms. There is no depression underlying the symptoms: it is the symptoms. If a person has the symptoms, they are depressed by definition. If this is so, why would you need a blood test to confirm what you can see with your own eyes? Suppose a person came to your office weeping, crying, filled with pathological guilt, and a host of neurovegetative symptoms anxious to kill himself/herself and end his/her misery. If there was a blood test for depression and it was negative, would you send the patient away untreated?

What if a person had an abnormal depression test, but was perfectly normal in terms of mood and behavior? Would you treat them? Do you see that this is really the only situation in which a blood test would be useful—to show an underlying risk for developing depression in someone who is normal? How accurate would such a test have to be to be useful? What if normal people with a value above a certain cut-off for BDNF or a cytokine had a 20% chance of getting depressed in the next two years? Would you pre-treat them? What if they had a 50% chance? Such a test would be statistically hugely powerful, but might still not be accurate enough for clinical use.

Per your question, the reason cardiac enzymes are so useful for diagnosing an MI is because you can't see an MI, you need some other way of identifying it, and because the enzymes are both specific and sensitive. They don't go up unless you've had an MI, and not much else makes them go up. Note also that the term "myocardial infarction" describes a state of observable tissue damage, not a group of symptoms. If depression similarly defined a simple form of brain damage, we might be better able to find such a simple test. However, depression is complicated in multiple ways. First, what we call depression is likely to reflect a whole passel of subtly different physical disorders. Second, in any given person, multiple pathways that interact in complicated ways are likely to be subtly abnormal, making it almost impossible that any given abnormality will provide a test proof positive of anything.

That's the first important question we'd want a blood test to answer. The second question invokes the hope that some type of physical measure will tell us ahead of time what specific types of treatment a given patient will respond to. This is not something that can be seen "with the naked eye," so obviously any such test would be hugely useful. Not surprisingly, therefore, many people have been searching for ways to predict individual response patterns, a pursuit fashionably called "individualized medicine." Approaches that have been explored include quantitative EEG, genetics, and neuroimaging. Several studies suggest that patients who fail selective serotonin reuptake inhibitors have higher levels of proinflammatory cytokines in their blood than do patients who respond,[1] which raises the possibility that these chemicals might provide guidance for predicting treatment response, but this has never been examined. In general, results for predictive methodologies that have been examined have not been very promising. In my opinion, it is unlikely that measuring any single chemical (or multiple chemicals) in the blood will ever provide an accurate enough picture of how to treat any given patient to be clinically useful, but I'm a pessimist and I might be wrong.

Finally, a blood test for depression would be extremely useful if it could tell us what was likely to happen to particular patients in the future over and above what we can predict from symptoms and disease course to date. For example, wouldn't it be useful to have a test that could take two patients who had both responded to an antidepressant and identify one who will do well long-term and the other who will relapse quickly despite appearing identical symptomatically to the first patient? As it turns out there is a biological test that has shown significant promise in this regard, but it is not a simple blood test. The dexamethasone-corticotrophin-releasing hormone stimulation (DEX-CRH) test provides a measure of how sensitive the hypothalamic-pituitary-adrenal (HPA) axis is to the inhibitory effects of cortisol.

Patients with depression tend to be less sensitive to this inhibitory feedback than normal individuals, which is also the basis for the more famous dexamethasone suppression test and works on the same principal.[2] Several studies have shown that patients who are resistant to cortisol and who do not become sensitive following antidepressant treatment are much more likely than others to relapse, regardless of any symptomatic improvement.[3,4] There are a couple of caveats. First, the association is not one-to-one, so it is not an exact measure of risk. And second, the test requires a number of hours, multiple blood draws, and the administration of CRH, making it cumbersome. Whether other simpler blood measures will be shown to have prognostic value following treatment is an open question. In general, treatment corrects (or improves) biochemical abnormalities when it works, but we know significantly less about the increased risk for relapse posed by any particular chemical not normalizing.

In summary, I think that diagnostic blood tests will probably remain in the realm of the unicorns; tests for individualizing treatment are being actively investigated, but face multiple challenges in terms of ever being clinically useful enough to justify their inclusion in our armamentarium. Tests to identify long-term outcomes may, in fact, be the most promising first use for biological tests.

REFERENCES
1. Miller AH, Maletic V, Raison CL. Inflammation and its discontents: the role of cytokines in the pathophysiology of major depression. *Biol Psychiatry.* 2009;65(9):732-741.
2. Raison CL, Miller AH. When not enough is too much: the role of insufficient glucocorticoid signaling in the pathophysiology of stress-related disorders. *Am J Psychiatry.* 2003;160(9):1554-1565.
3. Zobel AW, Nickel T, Sonntag A, et al. Cortisol response in the combined dexamethasone/CRH test as predictor of relapse in patients with remitted depression. A prospective study. *J Psychiatr Res.* 2001;35(2):83-94.
4. Ising M, Horstmann S, Kloiber S, et al. Combined dexamethasone/corticotropin releasing hormone test predicts treatment response in major depression - a potential biomarker? *Biol Psychiatry.* 2007;62(1):47-54.

Depression and Thermoregulation

QUESTION: "Would you try fever therapy for inflammation/depression (i.e., sauna 'fibrogenics')?"

Charles Raison, MD:

This question is insightful, but it also demonstrates a very common confusion about two very distinct states—in this case hyperthermia and fever. Before I answer the question, let's do a quick review of hyperthermia. Then we'll talk about what fever is, what causes it, and what it is for.

Let's start with the sauna. Many of us find saunas, steam rooms, and hot tubs to be relaxing. But let's think for a moment about what they do. Each of us has the equivalent of a thermostat in our brain and spinal cord. Most of the apparatus resides in the hypothalamus, a brain region essential for the brain's control of all types of circadian rhythms.[1] This thermostat likes to keep the body at an average temperature of 37° C or 98.6° F. But the thermostat has its own daily rhythm that keeps the body cooler at night during sleep and warmer during the day during wakefulness, with a peak temperature in the late afternoon/early evening.

What happens when you step into the sauna? Suddenly, you are in an extremely hot environment that begins to warm the body. Like the thermostat in your house, the thermostat in your brain wastes no time in responding and trying to keep the temperature at 37° C. A hot day causes the thermostat in your house to turn on the air conditioning. The heat of the sauna causes your bodily thermostat to do what amounts to the same thing. In the case of the body, the equivalent of air conditioning is all the processes that lower body temperature. These include sweating (the equivalent of a swamp cooler), bringing blood to the skin to be cooled, and driving the brain to change our behavior. If we weren't naked already, we'd get rid of as many clothes as possible, and we'd stretch out catawampus. Sitting in a sauna is a classic example of hyperthermia: we are hotter than our thermostat wants us to be, and our body is in active heat shedding mode.

The first thing to say about fever is that it is exactly the opposite of the sauna experience. Fever is best defined as a condition in which the setting of our thermostat is increased. Think of what happens when you get the flu. As the illness comes on, you begin to feel chilled even in a warm environment. Why? Because your body is responding to the virus, but upping the thermostat. Your body is sitting at 37° C, but your thermostat has now been reset to 38° C. Suddenly, you feel very hypothermic and crave to get warmer. In this way, getting a fever is like being out on a very cold day. In such a circumstance although your thermostat is at 37° C, you are losing so much heat to the environment that your body is below that temperature. That is what it means to feel cold: to have a body with a temperature below what the thermostat wants. In response to this, you do everything you can to increase your core temperature. You shiver uncontrollably; you curl up into a ball; you pile on the covers. Although not under conscious control, you also divert blood away from the periphery to the center of your body to keep it warmer and to reduce heat loss. You activate metabolic pathways to increase heat production. Urination increases to lose water, because water is more difficult than tissue to heat. Your body temperature begins to rise until it matches the higher thermoregulatory set point, and then you feel more normal. Take an aspirin, which blocks inflammation and thus lowers the set point, and all of a sudden you feel hot. Now your temperature is above the set point, and you are in a situation analogous to the sauna. You begin to sweat; you kick off the covers; and you stretch out on the bed.

With this introduction, let me cut to the chase. Significant data suggest that depression is associated with an increase in the thermoregulatory set point[2-5]; whereas states of emotional resilience are characterized by the ability to tolerate cold,[6-9] which occurs when the set point is lowered. Depression is like a fever, and well-being is a little bit more like the sauna. If you've never heard this before, don't feel uninformed. The connection between major depression and thermoregulation is one of the least known areas in the biology of mood disorders. Nonetheless, a number of studies have shown that medically healthy individuals with depression have elevated body temperatures compared to people without depression.[2-5] My favorite study was done by an old mentor of mine, Marty Szuba (before he tragically died of pancreatic cancer as a young man). He measured core body temperature in a group of individuals with and without depression and showed, as had others before him, that people with depression had elevated body temperatures across the entire circadian cycle.[2] Most remarkably, he then treated patients with depression with electroconvulsive therapy (ECT), and when they had remitted, he re-measured their core body temperatures. In remission, their body temperatures were indistinguishable from the control participants. In other words, treatment with ECT had lowered the thermoregulatory set point—a little like "electric aspirin." And, indeed, many studies show that antidepressants (but not traditional antipsychotics) lower brain and body temperature.

Why should individuals with depression be mildly febrile? The most likely answer to this question is that depression is often characterized by inflammatory changes that are also seen in response to infection.[10] Indeed, many studies now suggest that medically healthy individuals with depression have elevated levels of many inflammatory chemicals, any of which has the ability to increase the thermoregulatory set point. Where does the inflammation come from? No one knows for sure, but it is fascinating that psychological stress robustly activates inflammation, and does so more in people with depression than in people without depression.[11] If you are following this line of reasoning you might predict that psychological stress should also increase body temperature, and you'd be right. Although not much discussed, the phenomenon of "psychogenic fever" has been known for years.[12]

But the world is a complicated place. Many studies show that chronic exposure to inflammatory chemicals (called cytokines) produces depression.[10] Studies
in animals and humans suggest that before the depression sets in, inflammation
might actually have antidepressant properties. In this regard, the classic study
was done a decade or more ago by Bauer and colleagues.[13] They enrolled a small
group of severely depressed patients and injected them with a substance called
endotoxin, which produces an intense inflammatory response in humans. After
endotoxin administration, all of the patients developed a fever and felt "a little
punk," to quote my grandmother. But the next day, most of the patients had a
remission in their depressive symptoms that lasted until they fell asleep. The improvement in depressive symptoms correlated with how high cytokine levels rose,
and how disrupted sleep became in response. In this regard, we've known for years
that suppression of REM sleep has an acute antidepressant effect, and cytokines
(at high levels) disrupt REM sleep. So it appears that the acute antidepressant effects of inflammation in these patients with depression resulted from the ability of
cytokines to suppress REM sleep. As with sleep disruption treatment in general,
because the effects are transient, making patients with depression sick to treat
their mood disorder has never caught on, and remains a scientific curiosity.

On the other hand, I've suspected for years that strategies for lowering the
thermoregulatory set point might have real therapeutic potential, although this
hunch is only based on circumstantial evidence. Many studies have shown that
cold tolerance is associated with emotional well-being, whereas cold intolerance
is associated with anxiety and related constructs such as neuroticism. It turns out
that anyone can lower their set point by spending a lot of time out in the cold.
Studies show, for example, that athletes in cold climates become much more able
to tolerate cold temperatures at the end of the winter than at the beginning.[14] This
toleration is a direct reflection of a lowering of the set point, because doing this
makes colder temperatures feel "normal." Certain classes of people have been able
to spectacularly lower their set point such that they can tolerate temperatures that
would kill most people. Examples of these people include the Ama divers of Japan
and aborigines of Australia.[15] My favorite example, however, are Tibetan Buddhist monks who practice a form of meditation called tummo. This meditation is
practiced to produce profound and stable states of bliss—which to my mind really
highlights the link between body temperature and mood. Traditionally, to prove
their prowess, tummo practitioners perform remarkable feats of cold tolerance,
such as laying out all night in subfreezing temperatures without more than a sheet
for cover.[16] One of these rituals was actually filmed many years ago, providing very
strong evidence that tummo does indeed profoundly lower the thermoregulatory
set point.

So, a long answer to a short question.

REFERENCES

1. Rothwell NJ. CNS regulation of thermogenesis. *Crit Rev Neurobiol.* 1994;8(1-2):1-10.
2. Szuba MP, Guze BH, Baxter LR Jr. Electroconvulsive therapy increases circadian amplitude and low-

ers core body temperature in depressed subjects. *Biol Psychiatry*. 1997;42(12):1130-1137.

3. Avery DH, Wildschiodtz G, Smallwood RG, et al. REM latency and core temperature relationships in primary depression. *Acta Psychiatr Scand*. 1986;74(3):269-280.

4. Avery DH, Shah SH, Eder DN, Wildschiodtz G. Nocturnal sweating and temperature in depression. *Acta Psychiatr Scand*. 1999;100(4):295-301.

5. Arbisi PA, Depue RA, Krauss S, et al. Heat-loss response to a thermal challenge in seasonal affective disorder. *Psychiatry Res*. 1994;52(2):199-214.

6. Huber A, Suman AL, Biasi G, Carli G. Alexithymia in fibromyalgia syndrome: associations with ongoing pain, experimental pain sensitivity and illness behavior. *J Psychosom Res*. 2009;66(5):425-433.

7. Lu Q, Tsao JC, Myers CD, et al. Coping predictors of children's laboratory-induced pain tolerance, intensity, and unpleasantness. *J Pain*. 2007;8(9):708-717.

8. Uman LS, Stewart SH, Watt MC, Johnston A. Differences in high and low anxiety sensitive women's responses to a laboratory-based cold pressor task. *Cogn Behav Ther*. 2006;35(4):189-197.

9. Shiomi K. Relations of pain threshold and pain tolerance in cold water with scores on Maudsley Personality Inventory and Manifest Anxiety Scale. *Percept Mot Skills*. 1978;47(3 Pt 2):1155-1158.

10. Miller AH, Maletic V, Raison CL. Inflammation and its discontents: the role of cytokines in the pathophysiology of major depression. *Biol Psychiatry*. 2009;65(9):732-741.

11. Pace TW, Mletzko TC, Alagbe O, et al. Increased stress-induced inflammatory responses in male patients with major depression and increased early life stress. *Am J Psychiatry*. 2006;163(9):1630-1633.

12. Oka T, Oka K, Hori T. Mechanisms and mediators of psychological stress-induced rise in core temperature. *Psychosom Med*. 2001;63(3):476-486.

13. Bauer J, Hohagen F, Gimmel E, et al. Induction of cytokine synthesis and fever suppresses REM sleep and improves mood in patients with major depression. *Biol Psychiatry*. 1995;38(9):611-621.

14. Lane AM, Terry PC, Stevens MJ, et al. Mood responses to athletic performance in extreme environments. *J Sports Sci*. 2004;22(10):886-897; discussion 897.

15. Park YS, Rennie DW, Lee IS, et al. Time course of deacclimatization to cold water immersion in Korean women divers. *J Appl Physiol*. 1983;54(6):1708-1716.

16. Benson H, Lehmann JW, Malhotra MS, et al. Body temperature changes during the practice of g Tum-mo yoga. *Nature*. 1982;295(5846):234-236.

Body Temperature, Meditation, and Depression

QUESTION: "Please follow up on your comment about the relationship between body temperature, meditation, and depression."

Charles Raison, MD:

This seems like an odd query about an obscure topic, so it might surprise my readers to know that I owe my entire research career in mind-body medicine/psychoneuroimmunology to my "once upon a time" obsession with answering this very question. Although a little unorthodox, allow me to recount the narrative of my pursuit of an answer as a way of bringing the potential importance of the links between body temperature, meditation, and depression to life.

In the fall of 1997, I was working full-time as a clinical psychiatrist, running (or co-running) several services in the UCLA hospital. I was going through a bit of an emotional rough patch in my life, and perhaps because of that vulnerability, had been powerfully moved by my recent discovery of Buddhist ideas about suffering in the world and how to overcome it. I've never been much of a meditator, but during that time, I was pretty consistent in attending teachings once a week at a Tibetan Buddhist center in town.

After one of these meditation sessions, it dawned on me that the old Tibetan Buddhist monk who served as master of the meditation center might make an outstanding speaker for Psychiatry Grand Rounds. However, when I approached the people who ran the business of the center, they demurred about this possibility, but immediately asked me—in something of a non sequitur—whether I would be willing to try to put together some type of big fund raising dinner at UCLA for the Dalai Lama's sister, who was one month away from appearing in Los Angeles on her first-ever book tour to garner money for the remarkable group of schools she oversaw for Tibetans in exile.

On a whim, and having no idea of the work that was going to be involved, I agreed to attempt this feat. What followed were four of the craziest weeks of my life. This experience was remarkable for a number of reasons, but primarily because of the access to Hollywood's elite that my mission instantly gave me. You'd be amazed how many rich, famous people in Los Angeles are either Buddhists or admirers of the Dalai Lama. The most important long-term outcome of all this was not meeting celebrities, but meeting and becoming friends with a most remarkable Tibetan gentleman named Lobsang Rapgay, who first introduced me to the mysteries of body temperature and meditation.

Lobsang was—and is—one of the most eloquent people on the planet when it comes to making complex ideas from Tibetan Buddhism understandable from the perspectives of physiology and psychology (he has a PhD in psychology and philosophy, and is a Tibetan medical doctor). We took to having dinner every

Monday night, during which time he taught me much of what I know about meditation in particular, and Tibetan Buddhism in general. It was during one of these dinners that he asked me if I'd ever heard about the practice of heat meditation or "inner fire" meditation. When I said I hadn't, he brought me back to his house and showed me two remarkable videos of tummo—as the practice is known in Tibetan—that rocked my world.

The videos had been shot by a team of cinematographers working with Herbert Benson of Harvard University, who is most famous as the author of *The Relaxation Response*. He had been invited, in the late 1970s, to study certain advanced forms of Tibetan Buddhist meditation by the Dalai Lama, and had found that several practitioners of tummo meditation had been able to induce remarkable (i.e., 15° F) increases in the skin temperature of their fingers and toes while doing the meditation, despite quite cool ambient temperatures.[1] While intriguing, these findings had none of the visual impact of two separate videos—one showing a group of monks stripping nearly naked and steam drying wet cold sheets on their bodies in freezing temperatures, and a second video showing a group of monks climbing up through the snow to sleep nearly naked overnight in sub-freezing temperatures high in the Himalayas.

I couldn't believe what I was seeing when Lobsang showed me these videos, but he assured me that advanced practitioners were indeed able to do these things, and that nothing magic was involved. His belief was that, through practice, the monks had been able to take considerable control of the metabolic activities of their bodies.

All this was interesting, but what sent me down the path of trying to research tummo was the fact that the point of the heat was to produce very stable states extremely positive emotion—bliss in the parlance of the practitioners. Why in God's name, I remember wondering, would anyone hit upon steam drying sheets through meditation as the best way to induce powerful positive emotions? And what did body temperature have to do with mood regulation?

Lobsang didn't have a scientific answer to these questions, but he went into a discourse that had a profound effect on my future work. He told me that from a tantric Buddhist perspective, the mind is a flighty thing. "We know this in our own experience," he said. "You get your mind in a place where it is feeling very good, and then one negative thought shoots in and it all comes down like a house of cards. This is why we say that trying to achieve enlightenment through mental means alone takes three kalpas [a kalpa is equal to 4,320,000,000 years!]. On the other hand, by exploiting the energy in the body, one can achieve enlightenment in a single lifetime. This is because the body can be put into conditions during which it produces extremely stable mental states that can then be used to withstand the vision of emptiness."

The notion that bodily processes could induce powerful and constant emotional states struck me as an insight in keeping with what I'd seen in severely manic patients, who had fixated—but maladaptive—euphoria, and who often ran their stress systems so hard that they would develop lethal catatonia.[2] I began to wonder if the tummo-practicing monks hadn't tapped into brain-body pathways important to mood disturbances of all kinds, and had learned to channel the resultant mood effects instead of being "ridden by them."

Lobsang Rapgay and I agreed on the spot that we would make an all-out effort to study advanced tummo practitioners from the perspective of Western physiology to understand what they are doing, with the idea that doing so might provide important insights into mind-body connections of direct consequence to mood disorders.

Thus began a year-long dive into every piece of research I could find on body temperature and mood. It turned out there was a great deal of relevant information, and it soon became clear to me that body temperature was largely regulated by pathways in the brain and body that were central players in the mammalian stress response, and that have been repeatedly associated with affect regulation in humans.[3] Although more complicated than this, to a first approximation when the body wants to raise its temperature, it activates stress systems, and when it wants to lower its temperature, it reduces stress system activity. Stress system activation also activates proinflammatory cytokines, which reliably induce fever by increasing the body's thermoregulatory set point. I began to wonder (almost certainly wrongly) whether tummo had something to do with the activation of stress and inflammatory systems.

From these observations one would predict that psychological stress should elevate body temperature, and it has been shown to do so in humans and in experimental animals.[4,5] In animals, the effect of stress on body temperature and inflammation can be blocked by inhibiting the sympathetic nervous system.[6] No one has ever looked—to my knowledge—at whether beta-blockers would lower fever during an infection in humans, but this would be a prediction. Given that stress is so powerful a risk factor for depression,[7] and given evidence that many patients with depression have increased sympathetic and inflammatory activity,[8] one might guess that depressed people demonstrate increased body temperature—and as I've commented in a previous blog—this turns out to be true.[9-11] Moreover, when treated, body temperature returns to normal![9]

Perhaps you can see how I got stuck for about a year around the fact that depression seemed to be associated with increases in exactly the systems you'd need increased to dry cold sheets, or sleep out all night naked, if you were a tummo practitioner? Or so I thought. The resolution to this question only came after I had relocated to Emory for the very purpose of trying to understand the physiology of tummo. Greg Berns, MD, world leader in neuroeconomics and all-around skeptic, had originally entreated the Emory department chair not to hire me based on the fact that I was clearly a "California flake" due to my meditation interests. However, with the passage of time, we became good friends. We got into a discussion of tummo one day by the hot tea machine in the department break room. At one moment of particular disagreement, he waved his arm toward the tea machine and said, "Anyone could dry wet sheets on their bodies on a cold day, this business with the monks is all smoke and mirrors!"

"Willing to place some money on that?" I asked. And with that, the contest was born to see if we—who had no tummo training whatsoever—could, in fact, dry wet sheets on our mostly naked bodies. Fortunately for our experiment, it was the dead of winter and the temperature was supposed to drop continuously over the ensuing week. During the following days, I would see Greg carrying around cups of hot liquid and studying the steam. Finally, a Saturday morning dawned clear and cold—28° F. At 7 AM, Greg and I, as well as neuroscientist and accomplished Zen practitioner Giuseppe Pagnoni, arrived at Greg's house, stripped to our swimsuits, and went out to the garage where fellow "researcher" Dave Purselle had soaked three cheap sheets in a pail of ice water. We took our best meditative positions, and wrapped the wet, ice-cold sheets around our shoulders. Almost immediately, the sheets began to steam profusely, and in fact, the evaporating water vapor gave us a sensation of warmth. "Nothing to it," Greg said triumphantly. "The trick would be to steam dry sheets on a hot humid day in summer!"

Thus, I came to realize that neither drying sheets nor lying out all night in the snow would require an increase in core body temperature. What it would require would be an ability to withstand cold without freezing to death and without shivering (monks who shivered lost the tummo competitions that were routinely held in old Tibet). Although we had steam dried sheets, we only lasted four minutes before uncontrollable shivering set in. This experience sent my thinking in all together different directions. How would one physiologically be able to withstand cold and not shiver?

The answer seems somewhat paradoxical at first, and that is to actually lower the body's thermoregulatory set point, which is exactly the opposite of what happens with fever. In fever, the set point goes up, a person feels freezing because of the difference between the high set point and their actual body temperature, and they do everything they can to get their temperature up to the set point (e.g., curl up in bed, shiver, pile on blankets, vasoconstrict).[12] Lower the thermoregulatory set point and you feel suddenly too hot. You sweat; you send blood to your skin to cool. I remember that I'd read years earlier that when tummo goes bad, it typically ends in an explosion of sweating,[13] which is exactly what would happen if it lowered the thermoregulatory set point.

Was it possible to lower the thermoregulatory set point, and thereby withstand cold conditions while keeping the extremities warm and not shivering? It turns out that the answer is yes. This phenomenon happens each winter to mail delivery people and construction workers who spend the season outdoors.[14] They end the season far more cold tolerant than they began it. It used to happen even more strikingly in a group of female Ama divers. These women dove in the north Pacific all year long for pearls without oxygen and without wet suits. Their ability to tolerate cold water exposure without shivering was remarkable, and was best at the end of the winter after a full season of cold water exposure.[15] Perhaps the world champions of lowering thermoregulatory set point were the Australian aborigines who were able to lower their body temperature to a remarkable degree, and thus tolerate sleeping naked overnight in cold conditions.[16,17]

This line of thinking has implications for mood. One would predict that a lowered thermoregulatory set point would be associated with protection against depression in particular, and with emotional resilience in general. To my knowledge, no one has ever tested this, but there are several lines of evidence consistent with it. For example, as I've already noted, antidepressants and electroconvulsive therapy lower body temperature,[9,18,19] which likely reflects a lowering of the set point. And cold tolerance has been shown to be associated with increased self-efficacy and decreased anxiety.[20,21] Another clear implication of this theory is that learning to tolerate cold temperatures might help mood disorders. It's interesting, in this regard, that people with major depression who sleep in a cooler environment have a more rapid improvement of symptoms than those who sleep in a room with warmer ambient temperature.[22] It is also interesting that antidepressants, and especially selective serotonin reuptake inhibitors, often make people sweat, which is a phenomenon consistent with the possibility that they induce a lowering of the thermoregulatory set point. People often discontinue the medications because of this side effect; I would predict that it should be associated with enhanced treatment response!

I am currently working with Christopher Lowry, a colleague at University of Colorado, to examine some of these ideas as they pertain to improving the treatment of depression.[23] But what of my dream of studying the great tummo masters? This is as close as I came. At Emory, I have done a series of compassion meditation studies with my good friend and colleague Lobsang Tenzin Negi. Like Lobsang Rapgay at UCLA, Lobsang Tenzin Negi shared my interest in studying tummo from a Western perspective. He runs a large monastery in Atlanta, which allows him to host many visiting Tibetan dignitaries. Several years ago, he hosted the abbot of one of the two monasteries best known for housing tummo masters. The abbot had a taste for steak, so we took him to a local Brazilian steakhouse. It was worth the price of admission just to see people's faces as I walked in with two fully robed Buddhist monks into that cathedral to beef.

After some gracious small talk, Lobsang and I brought the conversation around to the possibility of perhaps studying several of the monks at his monastery. His face was impassive in response, and he seemed to change the subject when he next spoke. "You know," he said, "one of our great tummo masters was touring through the lowlands of India recently. He had a very busy schedule and was always surrounded by people, so he was unable to practice his tummo to the degree that he was accustomed. One day, he and his attendants found themselves alone out in the country. The master slipped away from his attendants and found a quiet spot under a tree to practice tummo. He began his practice, and a short while later, a curious goat approached him and gazed at him in meditation."

After a pause I asked, "What happened to the goat?"

"He went blind from staring inappropriately at the master during practice," the abbot said.

I realized then and there that I was the goat, and that was the end of my career as a tummo researcher.

REFERENCES

1. Benson H, Lehmann JW, Malhotra MS, et al. Body temperature changes during the practice of g Tum-mo yoga. *Nature.* 1982;295(5846):234-236.
2. Tang CP, Leung CM, Ungvari GS, Leung WK. The syndrome of lethal catatonia. *Singapore Med J.* 1995;36(4):400-402.
3. Arancibia S, Rage F, Astier H, Tapia-Arancibia L. Neuroendocrine and autonomic mechanisms underlying thermoregulation in cold environment. *Neuroendocrinology.* 1996;64(4):257-267.
4. Marazziti D, Di Muro A, Castrogiovanni P. Psychological stress and body temperature changes in humans. *Physiol Behav.* 1992;52(2):393-395.
5. Zhou D, Kusnecov AW, Shurin MR, et al. Exposure to physical and psychological stressors elevates plasma interleukin 6: relationship to the activation of hypothalamic-pituitary-adrenal axis. *Endocrinology.* 1993;133(6):2523-2530.
6. Soszynski D, Kozak W, Conn CA, et al. Beta-adrenoceptor antagonists suppress elevation in body temperature and increase in plasma IL-6 in rats exposed to open field. *Neuroendocrinology.* 1996;63(5):459-467.
7. Kendler KS, Karkowski LM, Prescott CA. Causal relationship between stressful life events and the onset of major depression. *Am J Psychiatry.* 1999;156(6):837-841.
8. Miller AH, Maletic V, Raison CL. Inflammation and its discontents: the role of cytokines in the pathophysiology of major depression. *Biol Psychiatry.* 2009;65(9):732-741.
9. Szuba MP, Guze BH, Baxter LR Jr. Electroconvulsive therapy increases circadian amplitude and lowers core body temperature in depressed subjects. *Biol Psychiatry.* 1997;42(12):1130-1137.
10. Avery DH, Wildschiodtz G, Smallwood RG, et al. REM latency and core temperature relationships in primary depression. *Acta Psychiatr Scand.* 1986;74(3):269-280.
11. Souetre E, Salvati E, Wehr TA, et al. Twenty-four-hour profiles of body temperature and plasma TSH in bipolar patients during depression and during remission and in normal control subjects. *Am J Psychiatry.* 1988;145(9):1133-1137.
12. Saper CB. Neurobiological basis of fever. *Ann N Y Acad Sci.* 1998;856:90-94.
13. Yeshe T. *The Bliss of Inner Fire: Heart Practice of the Six Yogas of Naropa.* Boston: Wisdom Publications; 1998.
14. Rintamaki H. Human responses to cold. *Alaska Med.* 2007;49(2 suppl):29-31.
15. Hong SK. Pattern of cold adaptation in women divers of Korea (ama). *Fed Proc.* 1973;32(5):1614-1622.
16. Scholander PF, Hammel HT, Hart JS, et al. Cold adaptation in Australian aborigines. *J Appl Physiol.* 1958;13(2):211-218.
17. Bittel J. The different types of general cold adaptation in man. *Int J Sports Med.* 1992;13(suppl 1):S172-S176.
18. Duncan WC Jr, Johnson KA, Wehr TA. Antidepressant drug-induced hypothalamic cooling in Syrian hamsters. *Neuropsychopharmacology.* 1995;12(1):17-37.
19. Gao B, Duncan WC Jr, Wehr TA. Fluoxetine decreases brain temperature and REM sleep in Syrian hamsters. *Psychopharmacology* (Berl). 1992;106(3):321-329.
20. Mills WJ Jr, O'Malley J, Kappes B. Cold and freezing: a historical chronology of laboratory investigation and clinical experience. *Alaska Med.* 1993;35(1):89-116.
21. Uman LS, Stewart SH, Watt MC, Johnston A. Differences in high and low anxiety sensitive women's responses to a laboratory-based cold pressor task. *Cogn Behav Ther.* 2006;35(4):189-197.
22. Wehr TA. Manipulations of sleep and phototherapy: nonpharmacological alternatives in the treatment of depression. *Clin Neuropharmacol.* 1990;13(suppl 1):S54-S65.
23. Lowry CA, Lightman SL, Nutt DJ. That warm fuzzy feeling: brain serotonergic neurons and the regulation of emotion. *J Psychopharmacol.* 2009;23(4):392-400.

Sleep and Immune Function

QUESTION: "How are sleep and immune function connected?"

Vladimir Maletic, MS, MD:

Sleep is just one of the many rhythmic activities that are regulated by the function of our "internal clock." Hypothalamic suprachiasmatic nucleus (SCN) acts as our personal atomic clock; it is a nexus of pace-making network distributed throughout our brain and body. Secondary timekeepers in the brain include olfactory bulb, amygdala, and hippocampus. Metabolic processes and synthetic activity of liver and even skin cells are synchronized with the activity of SCN.[1,2] Over millennia of evolution, circadian coordination has become increasingly more complex to include regulation of sleep and wakefulness, hormonal secretion (e.g., cortisol and growth hormone), autonomic function, synthesis of neurotransmitters, temperature regulation, motoric activity, and even memory consolidation![1,2,3]

Melatonin—one of the circadian signaling molecules that helps entrain sleep to external light cycle—also has a prominent role in modulating immune function.[4] Conversely, inflammatory cytokines play a major role in sleep initiation.[5,6] Both are substantially influenced by "stress-modulators"—corticosteroids and norepinephrine.[7] Not surprisingly, some conditions characterized by hypothalamic-pituitary-adrenal axis and autonomic disturbance, such as major depressive disorder and chronic pain, tend also to be associated with significant sleep disturbance.[8] As a matter of fact, "flattening" of the cortisol curve in patients with depression is correlated not only with severity of depressive symptoms, but also impairment in sleep quality and reduction of total sleep time![9]

Recent studies have described elevation of inflammatory cytokines, mediators of innate immunity, during the sleep phase. Conversely, wakefulness is associated by greater activity of acquired immunity manifested by T- and B-lymphocytes and circulating antibodies. Under usual circumstances anti-inflammatory cytokines, such as interleukin-10 (IL-10), have lower levels during sleep and higher levels during the wake hours. Sleep deprivation creates a disturbance in immune regulation: elevation of proinflammatory cytokines (IL-6, IL-12) in the early morning hours with concomitant reduction of anti-inflammatory cytokines (IL-10).[10-13] This type of immune imbalance commonly leads to a sense of fatigue, sleepiness, body-aches, irritability, anxiety, depressed mood, and diminished concentration[12,14]; a state that may conjure up memories of mornings after busy call nights. Elevation of inflammatory cytokines is associated with autonomic disturbance and glucocorticoid receptor insensitivity, often leading to flattening of cortisol curve and functional corticoid insufficiency.[7,14]

No need to spell it out: sleep-immune disturbance is likely to become self-perpetuating. Based on this description, one would expect to find association between sleep and circadian disorders and multiple medical conditions related to increased inflammatory response and immune dysregulation. This is unfortunately true: insomnia and circadian disorders are commonly associated with substantially elevated risk of cardiovascular disease, metabolic syndrome, type 2 diabetes, obesity, and even cancer.[15,16] Recent scientific discoveries, like the ones connecting somatic illness with sleep-immune disorders, have virtually rendered Cartesian mind-body duality obsolete.

REFERENCES

1. Mendoza J, Challet E. Brain clocks: from the suprachiasmatic nuclei to a cerebral network. *Neuroscientist*. 2009;15(5):477-488.
2. Gillette MU, Mitchell JW. Signaling in the suprachiasmatic nucleus: selectively responsive and integrative. *Cell Tissue Res*. 2002;309(1):99-107.
3. Buhr ED, Yoo SH, Takahashi JS. Temperature as a universal resetting cue for mammalian circadian oscillators. *Science*. 2010;330(6002):379-385.
4. Carrillo-Vico A, Guerrero JM, Lardone PJ, Reiter RJ. A review of the multiple actions of melatonin on the immune system. *Endocrine*. 2005;27(2):189-200.
5. Kapsimalis F, Basta M, Varouchakis G, et al. Cytokines and pathological sleep. *Sleep Med*. 2008;9(6):603-614.
6. Bryant PA, Trinder J, Curtis N. Sick and tired: Does sleep have a vital role in the immune system. *Nat Rev Immunol*. 2004;4(6):457-467.
7. Vgontzas AN, Chrousos GP. Sleep, the hypothalamic-pituitary-adrenal axis, and cytokines: multiple interactions and disturbances in sleep disorders. *Endocrinol Metab Clin North Am*. 2002;31(1):15-36.
8. Maletic V, Raison CL. Neurobiology of depression, fibromyalgia and neuropathic pain. *Front Biosci*. 2009;14:5291-5338.
9. Hsiao FH, Yang TT, Ho RT, et al. The self-perceived symptom distress and health-related conditions associated with morning to evening diurnal cortisol patterns in outpatients with major depressive disorder. *Psychoneuroendocrinology*. 2010;35(4):503-515.
10. Lange T, Dimitrov S, Born J. Effects of sleep and circadian rhythm on the human immune system. *Ann N Y Acad Sci*. 2010;1193:48-59.
11. Lange T, Dimitrov S, Fehm HL, Westermann J, Born J. Shift of monocyte function toward cellular immunity during sleep. *Arch Intern Med*. 2006;166(16):1695-1700.
12. Lorton D, Lubahn CL, Estus C, et al. Bidirectional communication between the brain and the immune system: implications for physiological sleep and disorders with disrupted sleep. *Neuroimmunomodulation*. 2006;13(5-6):357-374.
13. Burgos I, Richter L, Klein T, et al. Increased nocturnal interleukin-6 excretion in patients with primary insomnia: a pilot study. *Brain Behav Immun*. 2006;20(3):246-253.
14. Raison CL, Capuron L, Miller AH. Cytokines sing the blues : inflammation and the pathogenesis of depression. *Trends Immunol*. 2006;27(1):24-31.
15. Foster RG, Wulff K. The rhythm of rest and excess. *Nat Rev Neurosci*. 2005;6(5):407-414.
16. Wulff K, Gatti S, Wettstein JG, Foster RG. Sleep and circadian rhythm disruption in psychiatric and neurodegenerative disease. *Nat Rev Neurosci*. 2010;11(8):589-599.

Cortisol and Adrenal Fatigue in Our Patients

QUESTION: "Should we be measuring cortisol levels in our patients? What are your thoughts about the concept of adrenal fatigue?"

Charles Raison, MD:

Interestingly, if I had only a sentence to answer both these related questions, it would be a short one: "No." No, I do not think we should be measuring cortisol levels on a routine basis in any psychiatric condition. And no, I do not believe in the existence of adrenal fatigue as that term is commonly understood (i.e., a widespread condition of subclinical adrenal insufficiency that gives rise to a collection of nonspecific, and medically-unexplained symptoms, such as body aches, fatigue, nervousness, sleep disturbances, and digestive problems).

Why did I suggest that my negative answers to these questions might be interesting? Because if you had—for some esoteric reason—followed my research and academic writings, you would know that I am part of a research group that has spent over a decade working to establish the centrality of cortisol to a variety of psychiatric conditions. In this role, I have consistently maintained that psychiatric pathology is far more often the result of too little, not too much, cortisol signaling. Said differently, I am one of the rare folks in psychiatry who believes that cortisol is a good guy, not a bad guy.

This topic is so large and so important, but even this discussion will be inadequate, so let me start by referring you to a number of review articles on the topic (see references).[1-6]

To place the current discussion in context, we need to remember that in the early days of biological psychiatry, many studies showed that people with depression had very high levels of cortisol. In fact, the dexamethasone suppression test was initially employed, at least to some degree, as a means of separating out depression from Cushing's disease. These findings—combined with neurobiological understandings of the time—gave birth to an idea still current in many psychiatric circles known as the "glucocorticoid cascade hypothesis." This hypothesis proposes that an inability to cope with chronic stress causes a vicious cycle of excess glucocorticoid (i.e., cortisol) release and a subsequent compensatory downregulation of glucocorticoid receptors (GR) in the hippocampus, which further increases cortisol production, resulting in a feed-forward cascade of degeneration and disease.[7] In this model, cortisol is a major "bad guy" responsible for many of the pathological findings seen in major depression, especially loss of cortical volume in the hippocampus.

It is my read of the world's literature that 25 years of subsequent studies have mostly disconfirmed this hypothesis, and have done so by turning the "glucocorticoid cascade hypothesis" on its head. Instead of too much cortisol leading to downregulation of the GR, we and many others increasingly believe that the primary problem is downregulation or insensitivity of the GR, which then subsequently drives increased cortisol production as a compensatory—but ineffectual—means of attempting to get the "message through."[1] Note that a similar phenomenon is often observed in the early stages of type 2 diabetes, when reduced sensitivity of insulin receptors leads to compensatory increases in plasma insulin levels, which nonetheless are unable to adequately lower blood glucose levels.

From this perspective, the high levels of cortisol sometimes seen in depressed individuals reflect not too much cortisol, but too little! It is for this reason that we have argued strongly for the importance of not conflating hormone levels with hormone adequacy. Hormone levels are always only half the story, because they are always in a dynamic equilibrium with the amount and sensitivity of their receptors. Rather than thinking of hormones in isolation, therefore, we would do well to think about "hormonal signaling," which basically asks how well the biological signal for a given hormone is getting through given the current needs of body and brain.

A huge literature shows that environmental factors that increase the risk for depression also reduce the functional capacity of GR in both the brain and the immune system. In animal studies of early life stress, reduced GR functioning plays a central role in the development of adult behavior that resembles human depression. Michael Meaney and colleagues demonstrated that—in rats at least—the lifelong stress protective effects of "good mothering" were physiologically conferred by epigenetic processes that made the GR more sensitive—and hence more functional. More recently, epigenetic patterns consistent with reduced GR functioning in the hippocampus have been demonstrated in the postmortem brains of individuals who experienced documented child abuse,[8] consistent with the possibility that early adversity promotes depression—at least in part—not by causing too much glucocorticoid signaling—but by causing too little. Consonant with these findings, a recent study demonstrated that the ability of antidepressants to induce neurogenesis in the hippocampus was abolished when GR were blocked with RU486,[9] consistent with other studies suggesting that antidepressants work, at least in part, by making the brain more sensitive to cortisol.[10, 11]

Having warned against the dangers of equating hormone concentrations with signaling adequacy, it is, nonetheless, impossible to ignore the growing number of studies suggesting that many conditions associated with stress and symptoms caused by stress (such as exhaustion and bodily pain) are characterized by reduced levels of circulating cortisol.[12-14] These conditions include posttraumatic stress disorder (PTSD), chronic fatigue syndrome (CFS), and fibromyalgia. Even more convincing are studies showing that low levels of cortisol at the time of a traumatic incident predict the later development of PTSD.[15] A recent study that has been reported in the media, but is not yet published, followed up on these observations by showing that people treated with corticosterone immediately after a traumatic incident were less likely to later develop PTSD compared to people receiving placebo. Similarly, glucocorticoid administration has been shown to reduce chronic stress symptoms following prolonged stays in an intensive care unit,[16] and to increase people's ability to cope with stressful experiences (in this case, a standardized laboratory psychosocial stress test).[17] Finally, a recent animal study found that chronic corticosterone administration through adolescence led to increased hippocampal neurogenesis into early adulthood and reduced depressive-like behavior in response to stress.[18]

Hopefully, this quick review gives at least a glimpse of why I am so interested in the role of hypothalamic-pituitary-adrenal axis functioning in mood, anxiety, and pain/fatigue disorders, as well as why I believe that, in general, too little, rather than too much glucocorticoid signaling contributes to this welter of clinical problems. But still, we are left with a problem: because GR and cortisol levels exist in a seesaw relationship with each other, we are still left with the question of whether glucocorticoid signaling—considered as the sum of hormone levels plus receptor functionality—is really decreased in these conditions. What we need is some type of integrated read-out of glucocorticoid signaling to tell us how well the "full signal" is getting through.

Here is where inflammation comes to the rescue. Because cortisol is one of the most potent anti-inflammatory chemicals in the body, conditions associated with reduced glucocorticoid signaling should also be associated with increased inflammation, whether the reduced signaling occurs primarily at the level of the hormone (e.g., PTSD, CFS) or primarily at the level of the receptor (e.g., major depression). So what's the verdict?

Well, anyone following current scientific developments in psychiatry can hardly be unaware of the exploding database linking a wide range of mental disorders to increased inflammation.[19] This is a whole topic in itself; for current purposes, the point is that increasing data suggest that disorders associated with either low cortisol or reduced GR function tend to also be associated with inflammation, which we feel provides fairly strong evidence for true glucocorticoid inadequacy in these conditions.

REFERENCES

1. Raison CL, Miller AH. When not enough is too much: the role of insufficient glucocorticoid signaling in the pathophysiology of stress-related disorders. *Am J Psychiatry*. 2003;160(9):1554-1565.
2. Pace TW, Miller AH. Cytokines and glucocorticoid receptor signaling. Relevance to major depression. *Ann N Y Acad Sci*. 2009;1179:86-105.
3. Pace TW, Hu F, Miller AH. Cytokine-effects on glucocorticoid receptor function: relevance to glucocorticoid resistance and the pathophysiology and treatment of major depression. *Brain Behav Immun*. 2007;21(1):9-19.
4. Pariante CM, Miller AH. Glucocorticoid receptors in major depression: relevance to pathophysiology and treatment. *Biol Psychiatry*. 2001;49(5):391-404.
5. Holsboer F. The corticosteroid hypothesis of depression. *Neuropsychopharmacology*. 2000;23(5):477-501.
6. Yehuda R. Status of glucocorticoid alterations in post-traumatic stress disorder. *Ann N Y Acad Sci*. 2009;1179:56-69.
7. Sapolsky RM, Krey LC, McEwen BS. The neuroendocrinology of stress and aging: the glucocorticoid cascade hypothesis. *Endocr Rev*. 1986;7(3):284-301.

8. McGowan PO, Sasaki A, D'Alessio AC, et al. Epigenetic regulation of the glucocorticoid receptor in human brain associates with childhood abuse. *Nat Neurosci.* 2009;12(3):342-348.
9. Anacker C, Zunszain PA, Cattaneo A, et al. Antidepressants increase human hippocampal neurogenesis by activating the glucocorticoid receptor. *Mol Psychiatry.* 2011;[Epub ahead of print].
10. Pariante CM, Pearce BD, Pisell TL, Owens MJ, Miller AH. Steroid-independent translocation of the glucocorticoid receptor by the antidepressant desipramine. *Mol Pharmacol.* 1997;52(4):571-581.
11. Pariante CM, Makoff A, Lovestone S, et al. Antidepressants enhance glucocorticoid receptor function in vitro by modulating the membrane steroid transporters. *Br J Pharmacol.* 2001;134(6):1335-1343.
12. Van Den Eede F, Moorkens G, Van Houdenhove B, Cosyns P, Claes SJ. Hypothalamic-pituitary-adrenal axis function in chronic fatigue syndrome. *Neuropsychobiology.* 2007;55(2):112-120.
13. Tak LM, Rosmalen JG. Dysfunction of stress responsive systems as a risk factor for functional somatic syndromes. *J Psychosom Res.* 2010;68(5):461-468.
14. Bauer ME, Wieck A, Lopes RP, Teixeira AL, Grassi-Oliveira R. Interplay between neuroimmunoendocrine systems during post-traumatic stress disorder: a minireview. *Neuroimmunomodulation.* 2010;17(3):192-195.
15. Delahanty DL, Raimonde AJ, Spoonster E. Initial posttraumatic urinary cortisol levels predict subsequent PTSD symptoms in motor vehicle accident victims. *Biol Psychiatry.* 2000;48(9):940-947.
16. Schelling G, Kilger E, Roozendaal B, et al. Stress doses of hydrocortisone, traumatic memories, and symptoms of posttraumatic stress disorder in patients after cardiac surgery: a randomized study. *Biol Psychiatry.* 2004;55(6):627-633.
17. Het S, Wolf OT. Mood changes in response to psychosocial stress in healthy young women: effects of pretreatment with cortisol. *Behav Neurosci.* 2007;121(1):11-20.
18. Xu Z, Zhang Y, Hou B, et al. Chronic corticosterone administration from adolescence through early adulthood attenuates depression-like behaviors in mice. *J Affect Disord.* 2010;[Epub ahead of print].
19. Miller AH, Maletic V, Raison CL. Inflammation and its discontents: the role of cytokines in the pathophysiology of major depression. *Biol Psychiatry.* 2009;65(9):732-741.

Adverse Childhood Events and Risk of Autoimmune Diseases

QUESTION: "I was very intrigued by a slide you presented on Adverse Childhood Events and Future Risk of Autoimmune Disease and wondered if you could explain the study in more detail."

Jon W. Draud, MS, MD:

Thank you for a great question. This was an alarming paper to read. It pertains to a slide based on a paper written by Dube et al.[1] The aim of the study was to determine whether traumatic stress in childhood would increase the adult risk of developing autoimmune diseases. It was a retrospective study looking at 15,357 adult patients enrolled in an HMO and the Adverse Childhood Experiences (ACEs) Study. ACEs could have been childhood physical, emotional, or sexual abuse; witnessing domestic violence; and growing up in a household with substance abuse, mental illness, parental divorce, and/or an incarcerated household member. The total number of ACEs was then scored (0-8) and used as a measure of childhood stress. Patients were studied to see how many hospitalizations due to four rheumatic or 21 selected autoimmune diseases occurred.

The results were quite dramatic, I think, in that 64% reported at least one ACE, and the event rate per 10,000 patient years for first hospitalizations was 31.4 in women and 34.4 in men. Furthermore, first hospitalizations for any autoimmune disease increased as the number of ACEs increased.

We also know that the long-term effects of childhood traumatic stress will increase overall mental illness, suicide attempts, sexually transmitted disease, substance abuse, and even ischemic heart disease. Dube et al. found that the number of ACEs correlated with the likelihood of adult hospitalizations from autoimmune and rheumatic diseases, and the correlation was stronger in younger adults. This was the first study to demonstrate this correlation, and it is alarming to us as clinicians that events in childhood can presumably cause alterations of the immune system that manifest as illness decades later.

We know from our mind-body discussions that the nervous, immune, and endocrine systems are connected anatomically and functionally, and this is presumably the mechanism by which we explain the study. Essentially, the notion is that repeated "irritation" of the developing central nervous system (CNS) of children with excess corticosteroids and catecholamines may contribute to changes in the CNS and endocrine/immune functioning later in life.

Again, thank you for a great question focused on the study by Dube et al., which beautifully demonstrated the powerful interconnectedness of mind and body.

REFERENCE
1. Dube SR, Fairweather D, Pearson WS, et al. Cumulative childhood stress and autoimmune diseases in adults. *Psychosom Med.* 2009;71(2):243-250.

Chapter 3

COMORBID PSYCHIATRIC AND MEDICAL DISORDERS

Physical Illness in Patients with Recurrent Depression

QUESTION: "Please comment on the increased prevalence of physical disorders in patients with recurrent depression."

Jon W. Draud, MS, MD:

There have been many studies evaluating the prevalence of depression in those with medical illnesses, but few have examined the rates of physical illnesses in those with defined recurrent depression. Farmer et al.[1] studied a large case-control group evaluating physical illnesses in those with or without recurrent depression. They also measured body mass index (BMI) since many medical disorders are related to obesity.

Participants who were included had two or more episodes of major depression of at least moderate severity, and were interviewed by trained psychologists in graduate school. It was a relatively pure "depressive" sample in that participants were excluded if the depression was substance related secondary to medical illness, or if there was a family or personal history of schizophrenia or bipolar illness.

All participants were interviewed face-to-face, and *Diagnostic and Statistical Manual of Mental Disorders-IV* (*DSM-IV*) and *International Classification of Diseases-10* (*ICD-10*) criteria were used to measure depression. They were also asked about treatment for an array of medical conditions, including diabetes, epilepsy, asthma, hypertension, hypercholesterolemia, gastric ulcer disease, myocardial infarction, kidney or liver disease, rheumatoid arthritis, osteoarthritis, osteoporosis, rhinitis, hay fever, thyroid disease, and stroke.

BMI was also assessed and were classified as normal (BMI <25 kg/m²), overweight (BMI ≥25 kg/m² <30 kg/m²), or obese (BMI >30 kg/m²). Interestingly, 58% of controls versus 40% of participants with depression were of normal weight, and men with depression had significantly higher BMI values compared with men in the control group.

Hypertension, asthma, and osteoarthritis seemed to have the highest lifetime prevalence in participants with depression; whereas in the control group, asthma, hypertension, and hypercholesterolemia had the highest lifetime prevalence. In both groups, there was low prevalence of insulin-dependent diabetes, epilepsy, kidney disease, stroke, and liver disease.

All other disorders were reported as higher in participants with depression versus controls except kidney disease and insulin-dependent diabetes. Taken together, 14 overall physical disorders were shown to be more common in those with recurrent depression versus psychiatrically healthy controls. Interestingly, after controlling for BMI, depression was predictive mainly for the following six conditions: hypertension, asthma, gastric ulcer disease, rhinitis/hay fever, osteoarthritis, and thyroid disease.

Both women and men with depression had significantly higher BMI than controls, and one-fourth of women and men with depression were classified as obese. There are many possible reasons, including poor dietary habits, dysregulation of the hypothalamic-pituitary-adrenal (HPA) axis, and potential weight gain with antidepressant medications.

Many authors have hypothesized that activation of the HPA axis in these patients serves as a common mechanism by which catecholamines, cortisol, and cytokines in the periphery may predispose patients to greater medical illness burden.

Finally, these data and numerous other similar findings indicate that clinicians should keep a watchful eye for common medical conditions, including obesity, in our patients with chronic depression.

REFERENCE

1. Farmer A, Korszun A, Owen MJ, et al. Medical disorders in people with recurrent depression. *Br J Psychiatry*. 2008;192(5):351-355.

Anxiety, Depression, and Pain

QUESTION: "Several of my depressed patients report worsening of their pain symptoms with exacerbation of anxiety and depression. What is the connection between anxiety, depression, and pain?"

Vladimir Maletic, MS, MD:

The overlap of anxiety, depression, and pain is more a rule than an exception. Epidemiologic studies suggest that 30% to 60% of patients with depression also suffer from a painful condition. Presence of pain is a major predictor of depression and anxiety. A group of authors reported a type of "dose-response" relationship: the more bodily regions impacted by pain, the greater the prevalence of generalized anxiety disorder and major depressive disorder (MDD).[1] Furthermore, symptom severity in depression, anxiety, and sleep disorders predicted onset of chronic widespread pain in a 15-month prospective study.[2] It is becoming clear that the relationship between MDD, anxiety, and pain runs far below the surface.

Brain circuitry involved in regulation of emotions and stress response, to a significant degree, overlaps with components of the "pain matrix" involved in emotional and cognitive aspects of pain processing. Having in mind the evolutionary value of pain, stress, and emotions—mobilizing the organism to organize and execute an adaptive response—it would not be a surprise if nature, parsimoniously, selected overlapping pathways.[3]

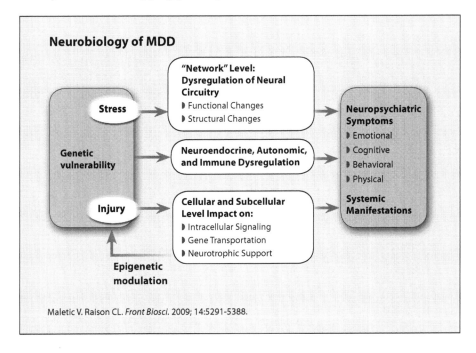

Maletic V. Raison CL. *Front Biosci.* 2009; 14:5291-5388.

There are important distinctions in the processing of pain, emotions, and stress response; pain sensory areas (thalamus, SI and SII) are less involved in the pathogenesis of depression and anxiety. There is a striking similarity regarding the involvement of limbic areas and paralimbic prefrontal cortex (amygdala, hippocampus, insula, anterior cingulate cortex [ACC], ventromedial prefrontal cortex [vmPFC]), as well as more "cognitive" and integrative areas, such as rostral ACC (rACC), dorsal ACC (dACC), dorsomedial PFC (dmPFC), and dorsolateral PFC (dlPFC).[4-6] Pain, anxiety, and depressed mood appear to have an overlapping capacity to engage autonomic, neuroendocrine, and neuroimmune components of stress response. MDD, anxiety disorders, and chronic pain conditions are all associated with altered sympathetic/parasympathetic balance, neuroendocrine disturbance, reflected in insufficient hypothalamic-pituitary-adrenal regulation, and enhanced proinflammatory response.[7,3] Given that these conditions have shared pathophysiological underpinnings, overlapping symptomatic manifestations should be no surprise. Full understanding of this "synergy" may have critical treatment implications.

REFERENCES

1. Manchikanti L, Pampati V, Beyer C, Damron K. Do number of pain conditions influence emotional status. *Pain Physician*. 2002;5(2):200-205.
2. Gupta A, Silman AJ, Ray D, et al. The role of psychosocial factors in predicting the onset of chronic widespread pain: results from a prospective population-based study. *Rheumatology (Oxford)*. 2007;46(4):666-671.
3. Maletic V, Raison CL. Neurobiology of depression, fibromyalgia and neuropathic pain. *Front Biosci*. 2009;14:5291-5338.
4. Fitzgerald PB, Laird AR, Maller J, Daskalakis ZJ. A meta-analytic study of changes in brain activation in depression. [Published erratum in *Hum Brain Mapp*. 2008;29(6):736.] *Hum Brain Mapp*. 2008;29(6):683-695.
5. Etkin A, Wager TD. Functional neuroimaging of anxiety: a meta-analysis of emotional processing in PTSD, social anxiety disorder, and specific phobia. *Am J Psychiatry*. 2007;164(10):1476-1488.
6. Baliki MN, Chialvo DR, Geha PY, et al. Chronic pain and the emotional brain: specific brain activity associated with spontaneous fluctuations of intensity of chronic back pain. *J Neurosci*. 2006;26(47):12165-12173.
7. Alesci S, Martinez PE, Kelkar S, et al. Major depression is associated with significant diurnal elevations in plasma interleukin-6 levels, a shift of its circadian rhythm, and loss of physiological complexity in its secretion: clinical implications. *J Clin Endocrinol Metab*. 2005;90(5):2522-2530.

Insomnia, Pain, and Depression

QUESTION: "I have noticed that my patients suffering from chronic insomnia, pain, and depression all have similar symptoms. Is this more than a coincidence?"

Vladimir Maletic, MS, MD:

Let's start our answer by considering a typical clinical scenario. Ms. X is a 43-year-old female complaining of feeling tired, sleepy, and "foggy." Her body is sore and achy "all over." She has little enthusiasm, limited ability to focus and complete tasks, and lacks appetite. Does Ms. X suffer from chronic pain, depression, fibromyalgia? Is she coming down with the flu? Or is Ms. X really a Dr. X who has just had a horrendous night on call? We really cannot be too sure, can we?

Sleep has an important role in immune modulation. It appears that innate immunity has its peak during the night, while acquired immunity tends to be allocated to wake hours.[1] We are not quite sure what is the adaptive value of this "division." Innate immunity taxes our metabolic capacities to convert our body into an inhospitable environment for the invading microbes.[2] It is mediated by peripheral mononuclear cells, inflammatory cytokines, chemokines, adhesion molecules, and prostaglandins. During the night there are fewer competing metabolically-intense processes. Therefore, it may be an optimal time for innate immunity.[1]

What happens if our nighttime sleep is disturbed? Individuals who do not sleep well are known to have a greater risk of cancer and less response to vaccines. It appears that lack of nighttime sleep shifts peak levels of inflammatory cytokines (such as interleukin [IL]-6) to morning hours. In the same context, anti-inflammatory cytokines (IL-10) have lower daytime levels.[1] In other words: our mornings become more inflammation-laden!

Neuropsychiatric symptoms commonly associated with elevated inflammation include: somnolence, fatigue, impaired concentration, irritability, anxiety, depressed mood, diminished appetite and sex drive, and lower pain threshold.[3] Sounds familiar? It should not come as a surprise then that insomnia is a predictor of widespread pain, depression, and anxiety.[3,4] Insomnia is also one of the most frequent residual symptoms of depression and a prognosticator of relapse, even in treatment responders.[5] If individuals afflicted with fibromyalgia do not sleep well, they are likely to have pain in more sites during the tender point exam the next day; stress will have a similar effect.[6] Fibromyalgia patients who also suffer from anxiety and depression show greater increase of inflammatory indicators (IL-8) than healthy controls or individuals who suffer from fibromyalgia alone.[7] A recent study found that sleep disturbance enhances the negative affect experienced by chronic pain sufferers.[8]

The relationship between insomnia, mood, and pain disorders is not casual, it is causal! These conditions are organically intertwined, sharing pathophysiological mechanisms such as neuroendocrine disturbance, altered autonomic regulation, and elevated inflammatory response.[3] Our patients would most benefit if we viewed insomnia as a bona fide pathological entity, not just as a symptom of another neuropsychiatric or general medical disorder. Screening psychiatric and pain patients for insomnia, especially women older than 45, followed by prompt and effective therapeutic intervention may significantly improve the quality of care.

REFERENCES

1. Lange T, Dimitrov S, Born J. Effects of sleep and circadian rhythm on the human immune system. *Ann N Y Acad Sci.* 2010;1193(1):48-59.
2. Miller AH, Maletic V, Raison CL. Inflammation and its discontents: the role of cytokines in the pathophysiology of major depression. *Biol Psychiatry.* 2009;65(9):732-741.
3. Maletic V, Raison CL. Neurobiology of depression, fibromyalgia and neuropathic pain. *Front Biosci.* 2009;14:5291-5338.
4. Gupta A, Silman AJ, Ray D, et al. The role of psychosocial factors in predicting the onset of chronic widespread pain: results from a prospective population-based study. *Rheumatology.* 2007;46(4):666-671.
5. Cho HJ, Lavretsky H, Olmstead R, et al. Sleep disturbance and depression recurrence in community-dwelling older adults: a prospective study. *Am J Psychiatry.* 2008;165(12):1543-1550.
6. Kamaleri Y, Natvig B, Ihlebaek CM, et al. Number of pain sites is associated with demographic, lifestyle, and health-related factors in the general population. *Eur J Pain.* 2008;12(6):742-748.
7. Bazzichi L, Rossi A, Massimetti G, et al. Cytokine patterns in fibromyalgia and their correlation with clinical manifestations. *Clin Exp Rheumatol.* 2007;25(2):225-230.
8. Hamilton NA, Catley D, Karlson C. Sleep and the affective response to stress and pain. *Health Psychol.* 2007;26(3):288-295.

Depression and Bone Loss

QUESTION: "Please comment on the connection between depression and bone loss."

Jon W. Draud, MS, MD:

This question relates to studies by Diem et al.[1] and Yirmiya et al.[2] First, Diem et al.[1] examined 4,177 women aged 69 and older from the Study of Osteoporotic Fractures. Depressive symptoms were measured by the Geriatric Depression Scale (GDS), and patients were categorized as depressed if their GDS score was ≥6 at the fourth examination. Bone mineral density (BMD) of the total hip and two subregions (femoral neck and trochanter) were measured at two exam points (fourth and sixth examinations) using Hologic scanners. Because it has been thought that some antidepressants have direct effects on bone metabolism, patients using antidepressants were excluded.

Overall, women with higher depression scores showed higher age-adjusted annualized percentage loss of bone density at the total hip than women with a GDS score ≤6. Similar findings occurred related to decreased bone density at the femoral neck, but not the trochanter. This is clinically significant because of the higher rates of fracture in elderly patients with depression. There are many possible reasons for the association, including decreased physical activity in elderly patients with depression, increased weight loss, increased smoking, and other medical illnesses like diabetes; chronic obstructive pulmonary disease and liver disease may also increase depression rates.

It is also known that patients with depression have impaired hypothalamic-pituitary-adrenal (HPA) axis functioning with elevated cortisol levels, and this may accelerate bone loss. Finally, there is upregulation of proinflammatory cytokines, such as tumor necrosis factor and interleukin-6, that may mediate bone resorption.

Ultimately, these are interesting data for us clinically and should prompt us to consider scanning bone densities carefully in our elderly patients with depression.

If we turn our attention to the Yirmiya et al.[2] study, the focus shifts to consider the impact of stress and stimulation of the sympathetic nervous system on bone loss. Estimates from several studies demonstrate 6% to 15% lower BMD in patients with depression versus controls. Whooley et al.[3] found that women with depression have a higher risk of osteoporotic fractures. Numerous authors have shown stressful life events to induce bone loss (e.g., Patterson-Buckendahl et al.,[4-6] Napal et al.[7]). The goal of the Yirmiya et al.[2] study was to establish the skeletal effects of chronic stress-induced depression.

Mice were exposed to chronic mild stress. They exhibited skeletal deficiencies and overall deficits in bone formation with increased bone resorption and a reduction in osteoblast numbers. Interestingly, antidepressant therapy administered to the mice (imipramine) prevented the behavioral changes from the stress and markedly decreased the overall bone loss. The depression triggered bone loss was associated with elevated norepinephrine levels in bone that could be blocked with propranolol, suggesting that the sympathetic nervous system has a role in the bone loss.

Additionally, we know that patients with depression have elevated cortisol levels and HPA dysregulation that may also have a role in the bone loss model presented here. Ultimately, the authors concluded that there exists a causative role for depression in skeletal deterioration that occurs secondary to the chronic mild stress, as shown by the fact that antidepressant treatment ameliorates the skeletal changes.

In conclusion, these findings do have clinical relevance for those of us treating elderly patients with depression and warns us that depression is a risk factor for osteoporosis and associated increase of fracture in patients with depression. This is another example of how the mind-body science principles demonstrate the amazing link between neuropsychiatric illnesses and peripheral bodily disease.

REFERENCES

1. Diem SJ, Blackwell TL, Stone KL, et al. Depressive symptoms and rates of bone loss at the hip in older women. *J Am Geriatr Soc.* 2007;55(6):824-831.
2. Yirmiya R, Goshen I, Bajayo A, et al. Depression induces bone loss through stimulation of the sympathetic nervous system. *Proc Natl Acad Sci U S A.* 2006;103(45):16876-16881.
3. Whooley MA, Kip KE, Cauley JA, et al. Depression, falls, and risk of fracture in older women. Study of Osteoporotic Fractures Research Group. *Arch Intern Med.* 1999;159(5):484-490.
4. Patterson-Buckendahl PE, Grindeland RE, Shakes DC, et al. Circulating osteocalcin in rats is inversely responsive to changes in corticosterone. *Am J Physiol.* 1988;254(5 Pt 2):R828-R833.
5. Patterson-Buckendahl P, Kvetnansky R, Fukuhara K, et al. Regulation of plasma osteocalcin by corticosterone and norepinephrine during restraint stress. *Bone.* 1995;17(5):467-472.
6. Patterson-Buckendahl P, Rusnak M, Fukuhara K, Kvetnansky R. Repeated immobilization stress reduces rat vertebral bone growth and osteocalcin. *Am J Physiol Regul Integr Comp Physiol.* 2001;280(1):R79-R86.
7. Napal J, Amado JA, Riancho JA, et al. Stress decreases the serum level of osteocalcin. *Bone Miner.* 1993;21(2):113-118.

Depression Following Myocardial Infarction

QUESTION: "Could you please comment further on the data presented relating to 'Survival Curves for Non-Depressed Versus Depressed Participants'?"

Jon W. Draud, MS, MD:

This is a great question and relates to a paper by Carney et al.[1] We have known that depression is a risk factor for mortality following an acute myocardial infarction (MI).[2-4]

However, most studies of depression and mortality post-MI have only followed patients for 12 months or less. Seeing as depression is generally chronic, Carney et al. postulated that the adverse effects may linger for many years, so they studied a cohort of patients for five years after MI. The other unique aspect of this study was that it was based on interview diagnosis of depression as opposed to traditional measures, which rely on self-reporting tools like Beck Depression Inventory (BDI) scores. Several studies have used self-report inventories to evaluate depression and MI.[5-8]

Patients in this study were enrolled if they scored ≥10 on the BDI and met *Diagnostic and Statistical Manual of Mental Disorders-IV* (*DSM-IV*) criteria for either major depression, or minor depression, or dysthymia based on a standard structured interview. The numbers were impressive versus previous studies, as 358 patients with depression and 408 patients without depression were enrolled.

The primary endpoint examined was all-cause mortality. Not surprisingly, the patients with depression were younger, had higher total cholesterol scores, were more likely to be female, and were more likely to be current smokers. Antidepressant use was not associated with mortality. The patients were followed for a median of 58 months and a total of 106 patients died over five years, including 44 of the patients without depression and 62 of the initially depressed patients.

The hazard ratio for all-cause mortality over the five years was 1.61 for either minor or major depression. The authors feel this is the largest study of patients with depression after MI by a structured interview protocol to date, as well as one of the longest follow-up periods examined.

The results confirm that depression is an independent risk factor for all-cause mortality after MI, and that major depression is worse than minor depression, hinting at a dose-response relationship between degree of depression and survival after MI.

One limitation of this study was that the effects of antidepressants were not measured. At baseline, 13% of patients with depression were taking medications. At six months, 36% were on antidepressants, but antidepressant use did not seem to predict subsequent mortality. However, overall use was not reliably documented.

Clinically, this leaves us as clinicians with a clear change to screen all patients vigorously for depression after MI. We clinicians have a strong sense that antidepressants are very helpful at "correcting" other disturbances along the mind-body continuum, and we have every reason to believe they would improve all-cause mortality after MI. Hopefully, future research will validate this theory.

REFERENCES

1. Carney RM, Freedland KE, Steinmeyer B, et al. Depression and five year survival following acute myocardial infarction: a prospective study. *J Affect Disord.* 2008;109(1-2):133-138.

2. Barth J, Schumacher M, Herrmann-Lingen C. Depression as a risk factor for mortality in patients with coronary heart disease: a meta-analysis. *Psychosom Med.* 2004;66(6):802-813.

3. Carney RM, Freedland KE. Depression, mortality, and medical comorbidity in patients with coronary heart disease. *Biol Psychiatry.* 2003;54(3):241-247.

4. van Melle JP, de Jonge P, Spijkerman TA, et al. Prognostic association of depression following myocardial infarction with mortality and cardiovascular events: a meta-analysis. *Psychosom Med.* 2004;66(6):814-822.

5. Lane D, Carroll D, Ring C, et al. In-hospital symptoms of depression do not predict mortality 3 years after myocardial infarction. *Int J Epidemiol.* 2002;31(6):1179-1182.

6. Lesperance F, Frasure-Smith N, Talajic M, Bourassa MG. Five-year risk of cardiac mortality in relation to initial severity and one-year changes in depression after myocardial infarction. *Circulation.* 2002;105(9):1049-1053.

7. Grace SL, Abbey SE, Kapral MK, et al. Effect of depression on five-year mortality after an acute coronary syndrome. *Am J Cardiol.* 2005;96(9):1179-1185.

8. Strik JJ, Denollet J, Lousberg R, Honig A. Comparing symptoms of depression and anxiety as predictors of cardiac events and increased health care consumption after myocardial infarction. *J Am Coll Cardiol.* 2003;42(10):1801-1807.

MDD and Comorbid Attention-Deficit/Hyperactivity Disorder

QUESTION: "I am uncertain of how to diagnose attention-deficit/hyperactivity disorder (ADHD) in my adult patients with major depression. Is this diagnosis even warranted in a patient with depression?"

Rakesh Jain, MD, MPH:

I completely understand your uncertainty. From a diagnostic perspective this is a challenging issue we often face. Matters are further complicated by the fact that from a *Diagnostic and Statistical Manual of Mental Disorders-IV* (*DSM-IV*) perspective, concentration difficulties are a shared symptom by both ADHD and major depressive disorder (MDD). Both of these disorders are high frequency disorders, both in society and in our clinics; hence, the question you have asked is one that confronts us on a daily basis.

Let's first examine the literature. Epidemiological studies do tell us that yes, indeed, these two disorders are frequent fellow travelers.[1-6] We also know that while each of these disorders individually cause a great deal of disability, their co-occurrence is quite disabling to our patients.[7-11] The data also point to this extremely important fact: while there are overlapping symptoms between MDD and ADHD, they are "stand alone" diagnoses that happen to love each other's company.[12,13] In other words, they often exist together, and that idealized outcomes depend heavily on us, the clinicians, being able to make an appropriate differential diagnosis.[14]

How is one to appropriately diagnose and treat ADHD in a patient with comorbid MDD?[15-18] I offer a three-step recommendation for you:

1. *Be suspicious, Be very suspicious!*
   Be aware that ADHD is a common comorbidity of MDD. Men and women, young and old—the risk exists in all populations.

2. *Screen. Verify. Confirm.*
   a. Always ask patients with MDD if they have a long-standing history of difficulties with attention, concentration, impulsivity, hyperactivity, etc.
   b. Ask if these difficulties exist only during a mood episode, or even outside of a mood episode (if it only occurs during mood episodes, this is not ADHD). Now, mood episodes can worsen the above difficulties, but the ADHD symptoms must have started before the age of seven (and can't be entirely explained by the major depression).
   c. Consider the use of screening tools, such as the Adult ADHD Self-

Report Scale (ASRS)[19-21] and ADHD Rating Scale (ADHD-RS).[22-24] I am a big fan of both of these instruments. The former is a WHO screening tool, while the later is based on *DSM-IV* symptoms, and I have found it useful for both screening and treatment response assessment.

d. Verify your positive or negative findings by obtaining collateral information (from spouses, significant others, friends, past educational or medical records, etc.).

e. Confirm your diagnosis using *DSM-IV* criteria. Some of the key elements of this are: onset of symptoms before age seven; presence of at least six out of nine symptoms in either/both of the inattentive items or the hyperactivity/impulsivity items; and impairment in at least two domains of functioning (school, home, social life), and that the symptoms are not entirely due to another psychiatric or medical or substance misuse cause.

3. Treat. Watch. Recalibrate.

Finally, in most instances it is appropriate to treat the major depression first as optimally as possible, and then reassess for the progression of the patient's ADHD symptoms and impairment. If they are indeed present and impairing, biopsychosocial treatment of the ADHD is highly appropriate. This will often include behavioral and psychological help, and if needed, appropriate pharmacotherapy of ADHD.

As most likely have astutely noted, there is no proscription in *DSM-IV* from making a comorbid diagnosis. In fact, we are encouraged by the extant literature to make such multiple diagnoses if the evidence for it exists.

REFERENCES

1. McIntyre RS, Kennedy SH, Soczynska JK, et al. Attention-deficit/hyperactivity disorder in adults with bipolar disorder or major depressive disorder: results from the international mood disorders collaborative project. *Prim Care Companion J Clin Psychiatry.* 2010;12(3).
2. Waite R, Tran M. ADHD among a cohort of ethnic minority women. *Women Health.* 2010;50(1):71-87.
3. Goodman D. Adult ADHD and comorbid depressive disorders: diagnostic challenges and treatment options. *CNS Spectr.* 2009;14(7 Suppl 6):5-7; discussion 13-4.
4. Biederman J, Monuteaux MC, Mick E, et al. Psychopathology in females with attention-deficit/hyperactivity disorder: a controlled, five-year prospective study. *Biol Psychiatry.* 2006;60(10):1098-1105.
5. McGough JJ, Smalley SL, McCracken JT, et al. Psychiatric comorbidity in adult attention deficit hyperactivity disorder: findings from multiplex families. *Am J Psychiatry.* 2005;162(9):1621-1627.
6. Kessler RC, Adler L, Barkley R, et al. The prevalence and correlates of adult ADHD in the United States: results from the National Comorbidity Survey Replication. *Am J Psychiatry.* 2006;163(4):716-723.
7. Park S, Cho MJ, Chang SM, et al. Prevalence, correlates, and comorbidities of adult ADHD symptoms in Korea: Results of the Korean epidemiologic catchment area study. *Psychiatry Res.* 2010;[Epub ahead of print].
8. Friedrichs B, Igl W, Larsson H, Larsson JO. Coexisting psychiatric problems and stressful life events in adults with symptoms of ADHD--A large Swedish population-based study of twins. *J Atten Disord.* 2010;[Epub ahead of print].
9. Biederman J, Ball SW, Monuteaux MC, et al. New insights into the comorbidity between ADHD and major depression in adolescent and young adult females. *J Am Acad Child Adolesc Psychiatry.*

2008;47(4):426-434.

10. de Graaf R, Kessler RC, Fayyad J, et al. The prevalence and effects of adult attention-deficit/hyperactivity disorder (ADHD) on the performance of workers: results from the WHO World Mental Health Survey Initiative. *Occup Environ Med.* 2008;65(12):835-842.

11. Birnbaum HG, Kessler RC, Lowe SW, et al. Costs of attention deficit-hyperactivity disorder (ADHD) in the US: excess costs of persons with ADHD and their family members in 2000. *Curr Med Res Opin.* 2005;21(2):195-206.

12. Quinn PO. Attention-deficit/hyperactivity disorder and its comorbidities in women and girls: an evolving picture. *Curr Psychiatry Rep.* 2008;10(5):419-423.

13. Fischer AG, Bau CH, Grevet EH, et al. The role of comorbid major depressive disorder in the clinical presentation of adult ADHD. *J Psychiatr Res.* 2007;41(12):991-996.

14. Babcock T, Ornstein CS. Comorbidity and its impact in adult patients with attention-deficit/hyperactivity disorder: a primary care perspective. *Postgrad Med.* 2009;121(3):73-82.

15. McIntosh D, Kutcher S, Binder C, et al. Adult ADHD and comorbid depression: A consensus-derived diagnostic algorithm for ADHD. *Neuropsychiatr Dis Treat.* 2009;5:137-150.

16. Antai-Otong D. The art of prescribing pharmacological management of adult ADHD: implications for psychiatric care. *Perspect Psychiatr Care.* 2008;44(3):196-201.

17. Newcorn JH, Weiss M, Stein MA. The complexity of ADHD: diagnosis and treatment of the adult patient with comorbidities. *CNS Spectr.* 2007;12(8 Suppl 12):1-14.

18. Diler RS, Daviss WB, Lopez A, et al. Differentiating major depressive disorder in youths with attention deficit hyperactivity disorder. *J Affect Disord.* 2007;102(1-3):125-130.

19. Kessler RC, Adler LA, Gruber MJ, et al. Validity of the World Health Organization Adult ADHD Self-Report Scale (ASRS) Screener in a representative sample of health plan members. *Int J Methods Psychiatr Res.* 2007;16(2):52-65.

20. Adler LA, Spencer T, Faraone SV, et al. Validity of pilot Adult ADHD Self- Report Scale (ASRS) to rate adult ADHD symptoms. *Ann Clin Psychiatry.* 2006;18(3):145-148.

21. Kessler RC, Adler L, Ames M, et al. The World Health Organization Adult ADHD Self-Report Scale (ASRS): a short screening scale for use in the general population. *Psychol Med.* 2005;35(2):245-256.

22. Szomlaiski N, Dyrborg J, Rasmussen H, et al. Validity and clinical feasibility of the ADHD rating scale (ADHD-RS) A Danish Nationwide Multicenter Study. *Acta Paediatr.* 2009;98(2):397-402.

23. Ohnishi M, Okada R, Tani I, et al. Japanese version of school form of the ADHD-RS: an evaluation of its reliability and validity. *Res Dev Disabil.* 2010;31(6):1305-1312.

24. Tani I, Okada R, Ohnishi M, et al. Japanese version of home form of the ADHD-RS: an evaluation of its reliability and validity. *Res Dev Disabil.* 2010;31(6):1426-1433.

Chapter 4

IMPLEMENTING AN INTEGRATIVE, MIND-BODY APPROACH TO THE TREATMENT OF MOOD DISORDERS

Five Traits of a Good Clinician

QUESTION: "What traits in us, the clinicians, affect outcomes in our depressed patients?"

Rakesh Jain, MD, MPH:

This is very well thought out question! We clinicians often talk about patient traits that affect depression outcomes, such as length of depression, number of previous episodes, etc. We also often talk about the capabilities of different pharmacologic and nonpharmacologic treatments, such as how quickly do the interventions work, how effective is it, how does it compare to previous therapies, etc. These are, of course, extremely important questions to ask. But, what we tend to under discuss is what about us, the clinicians, as a variable in affecting patient outcomes. What personal traits, habits, and belief systems in us, the clinicians, affect our patients' outcomes? Do you agree with me that this is often not discussed?

I am certain you have your own opinions on this issue, and I do too. A study by Schattner and colleagues[1] examined the issue of which physician traits do patients desire in a "good physician." Traits patients reported as highly desirable include professional expertise, patience and attentiveness, informing the patient, representing a patient's interests, being truthful, and respecting the patient's preferences.

I think your question genuinely demands I offer you my own personal thoughts and beliefs on this issue. I will leverage my experiences as a physician, times when I was personally a patient, and the experiences of my family members when they were patients. I believe there are at least five traits in a clinician that lead to a better outcome. If I were suffering from depression today and went to see a clinician, these are the five traits I would want to see in her/him:

A Genuine Empathizer – Someone who extends themselves to patients, not just because they are patients, but a fellow human being who's in pain. Many patients have reported the immediate comfort they feel with certain clinicians when they feel this genuine empathy emanate from the clinician.

A True Engager – Someone who wants to be a part of the solution to the patient's problems, someone who will engage the patient's support system in treatment, someone who realizes that depression is a tough disease to recover from on your own, and an engaged clinician is worth their weight in gold.

A Truly Honest Clinician – Someone who does not patronize their patients, nor do they harshly speak the truth. Someone who wisely wields the power that automatically comes with being a clinician. Honest, but not cruel. Honest, but not excessively blunt.

A Fine Educator – A clinician who recognizes that psychoeducation, if done well, is a gift that never stops giving. And, is willing to take the time to bequeath their patients the great gift of knowledge by talking to them, not ignoring them, educating them, and updating them to new developments in the treatment of depression.

A Realistic Optimist – A clinician who has a strong streak of optimism regarding their patient's outcomes, even when things are looking very dark. Patients and family members derive strength and hope from clinicians and a good clinician is never stingy in offering it to them, but in a realistic way.

These are my thoughts regarding clinician traits that lead to good outcomes for their patients.

REFERENCE

1. Schattner A, Rudin D, Jellin N. Good physicians from the perspective of their patients. *BMC Health Serv Res.* 2004;4(1):26.

Measuring Remission

QUESTION: "I know Remission is the goal of treatment in major depression, but how do I know when I am there?"

Rakesh Jain, MD, MPH:

This is a simple sounding question, but you clearly have articulated a concern in the field: How do we define remission, and how do we measure it? If we don't answer these questions, then remission remains just a highfalutin concept and not a reality for all of our patients. This would be unacceptable, of course. So let's have a heart-to-heart conversation regarding your very important question.

The most widely accepted definition of remission is the one used in most research studies, i.e., a patient achieving a score on the HAM-D-17 scale (17-item Hamilton Rating Scale for Depression).[1] This is a woefully inadequate definition as a score of 7 or less could very much indicate that there are still some symptoms of depression left over. Also, what about patient's functioning? Is that not as important as measuring symptoms of depression? The HAM-D-17 does not measure functional improvement. So, is it then appropriate to use only a score of 7 or less on this scale, a scale that does not even measure restored functioning as a measure of Remission? To top it off, use of scales and screeners in clinical practice is not a routine, and even the use of *Diagnostic and Statistical Manual of Mental Disorders-IV* (*DSM-IV*) criteria is not a routine clinical practice.[2,3]

We must, however, keep struggling with these issues as remission is such an important goal for our patients with major depression. Patients have a different perspective on remission too.[4] Substantial data support that remission is indeed the goal of treatment as it predicts so many things of value to a patient—better functioning, reduced risk of future relapses, better physical health, better outcomes for their children's mental health, less neurobiological impact of depression on the brain, among others.[5-7]

So, what is one to do? My suggestions can be broken into three points:

1. Certainly assess the patient clinically. Ask yourself: Are there clinically apparent *DSM-IV* symptoms of depression still present? Are there other symptoms of depression, such as irritability, physical aches and pains, ruminations, etc., present? Are comorbidities also "cleaned out"?[8] Is functioning restored to levels before the depression set in? Remember to assess for functioning in all three areas of human functioning—home, work, and social life. You may also want to assess for mental wellness as many, including myself, feel that the mere absence of depressive symptoms is not in itself an adequate measure of full remission. It's the presence of mental well-being and positive emotion, along with absence of all symptoms of depression, that constitute, in my mind, the kind of remis-

sion I would want if I were a patient and you were my clinician.[9,10]

2. Despite all of their shortcomings, the use of rating scales is truly, truly a great benefit to a clinical practice. I don't particularly like the HAM-D-17 for everyday clinical use. I would recommend the Patient Health Questionnaire (PHQ-9) for everyday clinical use.[11-14] There is even a two-item version (PHQ-2) that can be useful.[15] The PHQ-9 is easily found on the Internet, and it has demonstrated good psychometric properties in a variety of settings.[16] I found a great Web site that, with less than 15 seconds of providing registration information, you can access detailed information on the use of the PHQ-9 as well as copies of it for reproduction: www.depression-primarycare.org/clinicians/toolkits/materials/forms/phq9/.

3. Consider pushing yourself by not just focusing on whether any symptoms of depression are still present, but go beyond. Look for two other things: (i) What is my patient's level of functioning?[17-19] Is it optimized in all realms of human functioning—home, social, work; and (ii) Does my patient also possess, in addition to the absence of symptoms, the presence of positive affect symptoms,[20] such as optimism, happiness, hope, etc.?

This is a long answer to a seemingly simple question! However, it's such an important question that it deserved a full discussion.

REFERENCES
1. McIntyre R, Kennedy S, Bagby RM, Bakish D. Assessing full remission. *J Psychiatry Neurosci.* 2002;27(4):235-239.
2. Zimmerman M, McGlinchey JB. Why don't psychiatrists use scales to measure outcome when treating depressed patients? *J Clin Psychiatry.* 2008;69(12):1916-1919.
3. Zimmerman M, Galione J. Psychiatrists' and nonpsychiatrist physicians' reported use of the DSM-IV criteria for major depressive disorder. *J Clin Psychiatry.* 2010;71(3):235-238.
4. Zimmerman M, McGlinchey JB, Posternak MA, et al. How should remission from depression be defined? The depressed patient's perspective. *Am J Psychiatry.* 2006;163:148-50.
5. Trivedi MH, Hollander E, Nutt D, Blier P. Clinical evidence and potential neurobiological underpinnings of unresolved symptoms of depression. *J Clin Psychiatry.* 2008;69(2):246-258.
6. Maletic V, Raison CL. Neurobiology of depression, fibromyalgia and neuropathic pain. *Front Biosci.* 2009;14:5291-5338.
7. Krishnan V, Nestler EJ. The molecular neurobiology of depression. *Nature.* 2008;455(7215):894-902.
8. Greenlee A, Karp JF, Dew MA, et al. Anxiety impairs depression remission in partial responders during extended treatment in late-life. *Depress Anxiety.* 2010;27(5):451-456.
9. Achat H, Kawachi I, Spiro A 3rd, et al. Optimism and depression as predictors of physical and mental health functioning: the Normative Aging Study. *Ann Behav Med.* 2000;22(2):127-130.
10. Puskar KR, Sereika SM, Lamb J, et al. Optimism and its relationship to depression, coping, anger, and life events in rural adolescents. *Issues Ment Health Nurs.* 1999;20(2):115-130.
11. Kroenke K, Spitzer RL, Williams JB, Lowe B. The Patient Health Questionnaire Somatic, Anxiety, and Depressive Symptom Scales: a systematic review. *Gen Hosp Psychiatry.* 2010;32(4):345-359.
12. McMillan D, Gilbody S, Richards D. Defining successful treatment outcome in depression using the PHQ-9: A comparison of methods. *J Affect Disord.* 2010;[Epub ahead of print].
13. Malpass A, Shaw A, Kessler D, Sharp D. Concordance between PHQ-9 scores and patients' experiences of depression: a mixed methods study. *Br J Gen Pract.* 2010;60(575):231-238.

14. Furukawa TA. Assessment of mood: guides for clinicians. *J Psychosom Res*. 2010;68(6):581-589.
15. Arroll B, Goodyear-Smith F, Crengle S, et al. Validation of PHQ-2 and PHQ-9 to screen for major depression in the primary care population. *Ann Fam Med*. 2010;8(4):348-353.
16. Huang FY, Chung H, Kroenke K, et al. Using the Patient Health Questionnaire-9 to measure depression among racially and ethnically diverse primary care patients. *J Gen Intern Med*. 2006;21(6):547-552.
17. Klinkman MS. Assessing functional outcomes in clinical practice. *Am J Manag Care*. 2009;15(11 suppl):S335-S342.
18. Endicott J, Dorries KM. Functional outcomes in MDD: established and emerging assessment tools. *Am J Manag Care*. 2009;15(11 suppl):S328-S334.
19. Papakostas GI. Major depressive disorder: psychosocial impairment and key considerations in functional improvement. *Am J Manag Care*. 2009;15(11 suppl):S316-S321.
20. Slade M. Mental illness and well-being: the central importance of positive psychology and recovery approaches. *BMC Health Serv Res*. 2010;10:26.

Exercise and Depression

QUESTION: "As a mental health professional, what should I know about physical exercise when I am treating my patients with major depression?"

Rakesh Jain, MD, MPH:

Even though mental health professionals are known as "mind" clinicians, over the last decade, published studies have shown that we are the quintessential mind-body clinician. Emerging data on the use of physical exercise to treat depression powerfully reinforces this very message—that depression is a mind-body disease and treating it requires a mind-body approach.

We have long advocated physical exercise for our patients, but primarily for its clear and convincing positive benefits on physical health. You may be surprised to hear that the data on exercise's effects on mental health are very significant too! In fact, the data is so impressive that I am beginning to recommend it to every patient with a mood disorder I treat.

Let's first examine the data. Literally hundreds of pre-clinical studies on the effects of exercise on the brain have been conducted. Generally speaking, they reveal that regular exercise in animal models have shown increases in the size of multiple organs critical in mood regulation, such as the hippocampus, as well as an increase in brain-derived neurotrophic factor in specific brain regions. If you are interested in this topic, two articles I recommend you consider reading are from Pereira et al.[1] and Russo-Neustadt et al.[2]

There appears to be an additional benefit seen in animal studies—modulation of the hypothalamic-pituitary-adrenal (HPA) axis, which as we know, is crucial in stress management. If you are interested in reading more on the HPA axis modulation in animal models, I recommend two specific articles from Fediuc et al.[3] and Droste et al.[4]

There is a wealth of experimental and clinical data revealing positive effects on both the brain and mood in humans. Interestingly, exercise also appears to have a strong anti-inflammatory effect, which is an extra benefit to the individual with depression who exercises, as depression appears to have a large inflammatory component to it. Two studies worth reviewing to examine this experimental data in humans who exercise are from Pereira et al.[1] and Pedersen and Febbraio.[5]

The clinical trials data are actually quite impressive. Let's first examine a few individual studies, and then we will examine data from a meta-analysis.

One of the more impressive studies published relatively recently was conducted by Dunn et al.[6] Their data revealed that exercise as a therapy in patients with major depression was quite effective, but only if the patient exercised fairly rigorously and with regular frequency. Blumenthal and colleagues at Duke University published a study in 1999,[7] and then a follow-up study in 2007,[8] that compared the benefits of exercise with an established antidepressant. Exercise was nearly as effective as the antidepressant. Even more impressive, Blumenthal's studies revealed that exercise was effective in mildly as well as severely depressed patients. It also revealed that both supervised and home-based exercise were effective as depression interventions.

Now, a meta-analysis by Mead and colleagues[9] looked at this data recently, and it revealed some very interesting facts. It showed that exercise is effective in the young and old, male and female, and that regular exercise over weeks to months is more effective than infrequent exercise, and both aerobic and resistance training are helpful. I highly recommend you read this article.

In summary, it's time to start thinking about exercise as both a treatment for depression as well as an "add-on" recommendation for patients who are already on

Week 1		
My Goals for this Week		
Mood Scale 1 2 3 4 5 6 7 Very depressed Normal		PHQ-9 score Beginning of week: _____
MON Date _____	Activity: Mood Before 1 2 3 4 5 6 7	Duration After 1 2 3 4 5 6 7
TUES Date _____	Activity: Mood Before 1 2 3 4 5 6 7	Duration After 1 2 3 4 5 6 7
WED Date _____	Activity: Mood Before 1 2 3 4 5 6 7	Duration After 1 2 3 4 5 6 7
THUR Date _____	Activity: Mood Before 1 2 3 4 5 6 7	Duration After 1 2 3 4 5 6 7
FRI Date _____	Activity: Mood Before 1 2 3 4 5 6 7	Duration After 1 2 3 4 5 6 7
SAT Date _____	Activity: Mood Before 1 2 3 4 5 6 7	Duration After 1 2 3 4 5 6 7
SUN Date _____	Activity: Mood Before 1 2 3 4 5 6 7	Duration After 1 2 3 4 5 6 7
Inspiring quote here?		PHQ-9 score end of week: _____

antidepressant medications. Exercise appears to have a positive biopsychosocial impact on our patients who suffer from depression.

Clearly, a challenge in clinical practice is how to get patient adherence with our exercise recommendations. You perhaps have faced this situation in your practice as well. It appears that the use of structured, supervised exercise is helpful, as is the use of exercise logs to motivate/monitor our patients with depression. I have attached a copy of an exercise log I use in my practice—you are welcome to use it.

REFERENCES

1. Pereira AC, Huddleston DE, Brickman AM, et al. An in vivo correlate of exercise-induced neurogenesis in the adult dentate gyrus. *Proc Natl Acad Sci U S A.* 2007;104(13):5638-5643.
2. Russo-Neustadt AA, Alejandre H, Garcia C, et al. Hippocampal brain-derived neurotrophic factor expression following treatment with reboxetine, citalopram, and physical exercise. *Neuropsychopharmacology.* 2004;29(12):2189-2199.
3. Fediuc S, Campbell JE, Riddell MC. Effect of voluntary wheel running on circadian corticosterone release and on HPA axis responsiveness to restraint stress in Sprague-Dawley rats. *J Appl Physiol.* 2006;100(6):1867-1875.
4. Droste SK, Gesing A, Ulbricht S, et al. Effects of long-term voluntary exercise on the mouse hypothalamic-pituitary-adrenocortical axis. *Endocrinology.* 2003;144(7):3012-3023.
5. Pedersen BK, Febbraio MA. Muscle as an endocrine organ: focus on muscle-derived interleukin-6. *Physiol Rev.* 2008;88(4):1379-1406.
6. Dunn AL, Trivedi MH, Kampert JB, et al. Exercise treatment for depression: efficacy and dose response. *Am J Prev Med.* 2005;28(1):1-8.
7. Blumenthal JA, Babyak MA, et al. Effects of exercise training on older patients with major depression. *Arch Intern Med.* 1999; 159(19):2349-2356.
8. Blumenthal JA, Babyak MA, Doraiswamy PM, et al. Exercise and pharmacotherapy in the treatment of major depressive disorder. *Psychosom Med.* 2007;69(7):587-596.
9. Mead GE, Morley W, Campbell P, et al. Exercise for depression. *Cochrane Database Syst Rev.* 2008;(4):CD004366.

Omega-3 Fatty Acids for Mood Disorders

QUESTION: "Any data yet on using 'immune stabilizing' vitamin/dietary supplements as antidepressant adjuncts?"

Charles Raison, MD:

This is a great question, and the short answer is that there are all sorts of data around this issue, especially regarding the use of omega-3 fatty acids for mood disorders. As with all things psychiatric, the data are mixed with both positive and negative studies, but lest this dissuade us from seriously considering the potential benefits of these compounds, we would do well to remember that only 50% or so of all the antidepressant studies conducted over the years have beaten placebo.

Omega-3 fatty acids are not the only vitamin/dietary supplements with anti-inflammatory properties that might benefit depression.

As a quick primer, there are two types of polyunsaturated fatty acids—omega-3s and omega-6s.[1-3] Over the last 50 years in the west there has been a remarkable decline in the intake of omega-3s and a corresponding increase in omega-6 ingestion. Our diet is currently 20:1 omega-6 to omega-3, whereas an optimal balance is closer to 2:1. Omega-6s tend to increase inflammatory signaling, whereas omega-3s are anti-inflammatory and have other physiological effects likely to benefit depression. The challenge is that omega-3 fatty acids are essential—meaning the body cannot synthesize them and must obtain them from food sources. Good sources of omega-3s include krill, fatty fish, and flaxseed, hemp, canola, and walnut oils—none of which are consumed in any significant quantity by most of us.

Many, but not all, studies show that consumption of a diet rich in omega-3 fatty acids protects against depression, both at the individual and societal level.[1-5] There are several excellent reviews on this issue, most recently an excellent paper by a leader in the field of stress, inflammation, and depression, Janice Kiecolt-Glaser, PhD.[1] As I noted above there are multiple mechanisms by which omega-3s might benefit depression. They have been shown to increase vagal tone and dampen activation of a key inflammatory mediator nuclear factor-kappa-beta (NF-kB).[1] Just to put this in perspective, people with depression have reduced vagal tone and respond to stressors with increased production of NF-kB.[1,6-9] Given these data, one might expect people with depression to have reduced levels of omega-3s, and, indeed, a recent meta-analysis confirms that this is the case.[10]

There is a fairly respectable literature examining the efficacy of omega-3 fatty acids as treatment for both major depressive disorder (MDD) and bipolar disorder. A meta-analysis published in 2007 reported that, based on 10 randomized, placebo-controlled, double-blind studies, omega-3s (especially eicosapentaenoic acid [EPA]) appeared to improve symptoms of depression and bipolar disorder, although with the caveat that the studies were uneven and the meta-analysis was vulnerable to publication bias (i.e., negative studies don't get published).[11] A large recent study of EPA for depressive symptoms in perimenopausal females found effectiveness for women whose depression was not severe enough to qualify for MDD, but no difference from placebo in women with MDD.[12]

Recent interest has shifted somewhat from omega-3s as monotherapies to using these compounds as augmenting agents for traditional antidepressants. Here again the data are mixed, but perhaps promising. A small randomized study published in 2002 found that the addition of EPA to maintenance antidepressant therapy significantly lowered depressive symptom scores when compared to the addition of a placebo.[13] A large study published in Iran in 2008 found that the addition of EPA to fluoxetine in patients with MDD was significantly more effective than treatment with either EPA or fluoxetine alone.[14]

On the other hand, two studies using omega-3s as to augment antidepressants in medically-ill patients with MDD have reported negative results. Carney and colleagues randomized 122 patients with cardiovascular disease and MDD to either 50 mg of sertraline plus placebo or 50 mg of sertraline and a mixture of omega-3s. At the end of the study, response and remission rates were essentially identical between groups.[15] Similarly, a small study just out on PubMed found no difference between antidepressants plus EPA versus antidepressants plus placebo in patients with diabetes and MDD, although the study enrolled only 25 participants, making it highly vulnerable to type 2 diabetes as a result of being underpowered.[16]

What are we to make of all this? Well, let's put it this way—I take my flaxseed oil pills everyday, and I recommend the same for you. I think the data are strong enough given the benign nature of omega-3s to consider adding these to standard antidepressant treatment in patients with MDD.

REFERENCES
1. Kiecolt-Glaser JK. Stress, food, and inflammation: psychoneuroimmunology and nutrition at the cutting edge. *Psychosom Med.* 2010;72(4):365-369.
2. Logan AC. Omega-3 fatty acids and major depression: a primer for the mental health professional. *Lipids Health Dis.* 2004;3:25.
3. Freeman MP. Omega-3 fatty acids in major depressive disorder. *J Clin Psychiatry.* 2009;70(suppl 5):7-11.
4. Tanskanen A, Hibbeln JR, Tuomilehto J, et al. Fish consumption and depressive symptoms in the general population in Finland. *Psychiatr Serv.* 2001;52(4):529-531.
5. Dai J, Miller AH, Bremner JD, et al. Adherence to the mediterranean diet is inversely associated with circulating interleukin-6 among middle-aged men: a twin study. *Circulation.* 2008;117(2):169-175.
6. Udupa K, Sathyaprabha TN, Thirthalli J, et al. Alteration of cardiac autonomic functions in patients with major depression: a study using heart rate variability measures. *J Affect Disord.* 2007;100(1-3):137-141.
7. Rottenberg J, Clift A, Bolden S, Salomon K. RSA fluctuation in major depressive disorder. *Psychophysiology.* 2007;44(3):450-458.
8. Chambers AS, Allen JJ. Vagal tone as an indicator of treatment response in major depression. *Psychophysiology.* 2002;39(6):861-864.
9. Pace TW, Mletzko TC, Alagbe O, et al. Increased stress-induced inflammatory responses in male patients with major depression and increased early life stress. *Am J Psychiatry.* 2006;163(9):1630-1633.
10. Lin PY, Huang SY, Su KP. A Meta-Analytic Review of Polyunsaturated Fatty Acid Compositions in Pa-

tients with Depression. *Biol Psychiatry*. 2010;[Epub ahead of print].

11. Lin PY, Su KP. A meta-analytic review of double-blind, placebo-controlled trials of antidepressant efficacy of omega-3 fatty acids. *J Clin Psychiatry*. 2007;68(7):1056-1061.

12. Lucas M, Asselin G, Merette C, et al. Ethyl-eicosapentaenoic acid for the treatment of psychological distress and depressive symptoms in middle-aged women: a double-blind, placebo-controlled, randomized clinical trial. *Am J Clin Nutr*. 2009;89(2):641-651.

13. Nemets B, Stahl Z, Belmaker RH. Addition of omega-3 fatty acid to maintenance medication treatment for recurrent unipolar depressive disorder. *Am J Psychiatry*. 2002;159(3):477-479.

14. Jazayeri S, Tehrani-Doost M, Keshavarz SA, et al. Comparison of therapeutic effects of omega-3 fatty acid eicosapentaenoic acid and fluoxetine, separately and in combination, in major depressive disorder. *Aust N Z J Psychiatry*. 2008;42(3):192-198.

15. Carney RM, Freedland KE, Rubin EH, et al. Omega-3 augmentation of sertraline in treatment of depression in patients with coronary heart disease: a randomized controlled trial. *JAMA*. 2009;302(15):1651-1657.

16. Bot M, Pouwer F, Assies J, et al. Eicosapentaenoic acid as an add-on to antidepressant medication for co-morbid major depression in patients with diabetes mellitus: A randomized, double-blind placebo-controlled study. *J Affect Disord*. 2010;[Epub ahead of print].

Role of Vitamin D in Depression

QUESTION: "Please comment further on the roles of vitamin D and its role in depression."

Jon W. Draud, MS, MD:

This is an excellent question, and in my practice checking vitamin D levels has become a standard practice. It has amazed me over the past couple of years how common this deficiency is, and how correcting it can lead to mood improvements. That being said, what do we know about vitamin D and depression?

Nearly 20 years ago, Professor Walter E. Stumpf from the University of North Carolina predicted a major role for bright light therapy and vitamin D in psychiatry.[1] We now know that bright light (without vitamin D producing UVB [ultraviolet B]) does have positive effects on mood. The question remains whether vitamin D has a separate or complimentary effect on mood, as do the effects of bright light alone.

This gets to the concept of seasonal affective disorder (SAD). There is evidence dating to 1998 when researchers in Australia found that cholecalciferol at both 400 IU and 800 IU significantly improved affect when given to healthy individuals.[2] Forty-four participants were given drug versus placebo in the late winter for five days in a randomized double-blinded study. Results on a self-reported measure showed a full standard delineation of improvement in enhancement of positive affect. In 1999, Gloth and colleagues[3] found that 100,000 IU of vitamin D as a single dose was superior in improvement of depression scale measures compared to bright light therapy in patients with SAD. Other researchers have found healthy controls' average serum 25-hydroxyvitamin D levels of 46 ng/L versus depressed participants with levels averaging 37 ng/L.[4]

Many have theorized that the rates of depression have increased over the past 100 years and ongoing in part to vitamin D deficiency. Humans have decreased their sunlight exposure due to tall buildings, pollution, cars, clothing, and mostly indoor work habits. Low vitamin D status is a widespread problem in the United States.[5] Additionally, research by Wagner and Greer have indicated that vitamin D levels previously thought to be sufficient for good health are actually too low.[6]

There are numerous roles for vitamin D in disease states, including cognition, depression, osteoporosis, cancer, cardiovascular disease, and diabetes. Vitamin D receptors are found prominently in amygdala regions where behavior and emotions are regulated in the limbic system, and we believe that vitamin D can exert neuroprotective effects as well. Recently, Wilkins and colleagues[7] showed a link between low vitamin D levels, depression, and impaired cognition in older adults. Several other authors have shown a link between vitamin D levels and depression.[8-10] Martiny et al.[11] found that light therapy can improve depression along with antidepressants, which may, in part, be due to improved vitamin D synthesis with light therapy.

Results from various studies attempting to link vitamin D deficiency to depression have been equivocal, but recently 7,970 U.S. residents were studied in the Third National Health and Nutrition Examination Survey (NHANES III).[12] The participants were between the ages of 15 and 39, and we will discuss the study and results to help shed light on this issue. There was a significant association between depression and low vitamin D levels (odds ratio=1.85; P=0.021) when statistical analysis was corrected for sex, age, gender, race, poverty/income ratio, vitamin/mineral supplements, and medication use. The prevalence of suboptimal serum vitamin D concentration (≤75 nmol/L) was 50%; 20% were vitamin D deficient at <50 nmol/L and 30% were moderately deficient falling into the serum range of 50 to 75 nmol/L. Higher prevalence of vitamin D deficiency was found in women, non-Hispanic blacks, individuals with higher body mass index, individuals with lower income levels, and those living in the South and West regions and urban areas. This was surprising in terms of more deficiencies occurring in people in Southern regions, but this may have been due to the fact that NHANES III was conducted in the summer months, so maybe Northern participants would have been more disadvantaged if the study had been in the fall or winter.

In contrast, a recent study by Zhao et al.[13] found no significant association between vitamin D levels and depression.

We are still left with conflicting results, but I believe clinicians do not doubt this association and the strength of NHANES III is primarily study size—the largest cohort ever studied.

REFERENCES

1. Stumpf WE, Privette TH. Light, vitamin D and psychiatry. Role of 1,25 dihydroxyvitamin D3 (soltriol) in etiology and therapy of seasonal affective disorder and other mental processes. *Psychopharmacology* (Berl). 1989;97(3):285-294.
2. Lansdowne AT, Provost SC. Vitamin D3 enhances mood in healthy subjects during winter. *Psychopharmacology* (Berl). 1998;135(4):319-323.
3. Gloth FM 3rd, Alam W, Hollis B. Vitamin D vs broad spectrum phototherapy in the treatment of seasonal affective disorder. *J Nutr Health Aging*. 1999;3(1):5-7.
4. Schneider B, Weber B, Frensch A, Stein J, Fritz J. Vitamin D in schizophrenia, major depression and alcoholism. *J Neural Transm*. 2000;107(7):839-842.
5. Holick MF. High prevalence of vitamin D inadequacy and implications for health. *Mayo Clin Proc*. 2006;81(3):353-373.
6. Wagner CL, Greer FR; American Academy of Pediatrics Section on Breastfeeding; American Academy of Pediatrics Committee on Nutrition. Prevention of rickets and vitamin D deficiency in infants, children, and adolescents. *Pediatrics*. 2008;122(5):1142-1152.
7. Wilkins CH, Sheline YI, Roe CM, Birge SJ, Morris JC. Vitamin D deficiency is associated with low mood and worse cognitive performance in older adults. *Am J Geriatr Psychiatry*. 2006;14(12):1032-1040.
8. Jorde R, Waterloo K, Saleh F, Haug E, Svartberg J. Neuropsychological function in relation to serum parathyroid hormone and serum 25-hydroxyvitamin D levels. The Tromso study. *J Neurol*. 2006;253(4):464-470.
9. Jorde R, Sneve M, Figenschau Y, Svartberg J, Waterloo K. Effects of vitamin D supplementation on symptoms of depression in overweight and obese subjects: randomized double blind trial. *J Intern Med*. 2008;264(6):599-609.
10. Hoogendijk WJ, Lips P, Dik MG, et al. Depression is associated with decreased 25-hydroxyvitamin D

and increased parathyroid hormone levels in older adults. *Arch Gen Psychiatry*. 2008;65(5):508-512.

11. Martiny K, Lunde M, Unden M, Dam H, Bech P. Adjunctive bright light in non-seasonal major depression: results from clinician-rated depression scales. *Acta Psychiatr Scand*. 2005;112(2):117-125.

12. Ganji V, Milone C, Cody MM, McCarty F, Wang YT. Serum vitamin D concentrations are related to depression in young adult US population: the Third National Health and Nutrition Examination Survey. *Int Arch Med*. 2010;3:29.

13. Zhao G, Ford ES, Li C, Balluz LS. No associations between serum concentrations of 25-hydroxyvitamin D and parathyroid hormone and depression among US adults. *Br J Nutr*. 2010;104(11):1696-1702.

Seasonal Affective Disorder and Cognitive Functioning

QUESTION: "In a previous Q&A, you discussed vitamin D deficiency in depression. Could you further elaborate on seasonal affective disorder and cognitive functioning?"

Jon W. Draud, MS, MD:

This is a great question. The prevalence of seasonal affective disorder (SAD) seems to range from 1.4% in Florida to 9.7% in New Hampshire.[1] SAD was first described by Norman E. Rosenthal and colleagues at the National Institute of Mental Health in 1984.[2-4] Treatments range from light therapy and ionized-air administration to use of melatonin, as well as cognitive therapy and antidepressant pharmacotherapy. There is a great deal written about SAD, but I'd like to concentrate on the role of sunlight exposure and cognition.

A recent study examined the effects of sunlight exposure on cognitive function among patients with depression and patients without depression.[5] The rationale stems from the fact that suprachiasmatic nuclei (SCN) seem to link sunlight and mood as evidenced by serotonin and melatonin and their roles in depression. Cognitive functioning is involved in these same pathways and seems to be affected by sunlight.[6-8] The study examined 16,800 participants and posed the question of whether a close relationship existed with sunlight exposure and cognition in depressed versus non-depressed patients. The participants were 45 years and older and evenly distributed among 48 states, with 45% being male and 55% being female. A six-item cognitive questionnaire was used to measure cognition before and after sunlight exposure. The cognitive screener was divided into two parts: short-term recall and temporal orientation.

Participants with depression who had lower sunlight exposure had a statistically significantly higher level of cognitive impairments. Among non-depressed participants, sunlight exposure did not seem to affect cognition. The exposure was either a single day exposure or that given daily for a period of two weeks. There was, in fact, a dose-response relationship found between cognitive function and sunlight exposure (odds ratio=2.58; 95% confidence interval=1.43-6.69) such that lower levels of sunlight are linked to impaired cognition. This adds to the evidence that shows that lifestyle and environment have a profound effect on patients with SAD.

Data suggest that violent homicides, suicides, and aggression peak in late spring and are linked to climatic variables and sunlight.[9] It is now well-established that SAD depressive episodes are linked with the shorter daylight periods seen in winter.[10] This new evidence that sunlight exposure is linked with cognition in patients with depression gives further credence to the idea that the physiology giving rise to seasonal depression may also be involved in sunlight's effects on cognition. Leonard and Myint have even linked a lack of sunlight to altered serotonin levels, neurodegeneration, depression, cognitive changes, and even dementia.[11]

Environmental illumination has been shown to be important in both seasonal and non-seasonal depressions.[10,12,13] These theories linking seasonal cycles, depression, and cognition are based on circadian rhythmicity and the SCN.[3,14] The SCN are modulated by body temperature and physical activity, but specifically via light received by retinal sensors at wavelengths approximating 477 nanometers, which is close to "natural sunlight."[14] The SCN regulate numerous processes including the immune system, hormone systems, blood pressure, digestion, and sleep cycle and body temperature. Walker and Stickgold[15] have linked dysfunctional circadian rhythms with cognitive deficits, and Miller et al.[10] have shown that one of the SCN regulatory functions is to inhibit the pineal gland from converting serotonin to melatonin in the presence of daylight. Serotonin and melatonin have been implicated in many mental and cognitive disorders, including Alzheimer's disease, various sleep disorders, and Parkinson's disease.[16,17] Abnormalities in these systems have been shown to exist in bipolar disorder,[8] schizophrenia,[18] SAD,[16,19] and in those with no psychiatric illness.[20]

Furthermore, light seems to affect blood flow to brain. Dani et al.[21] have shown that cerebral flow improves in infants after phototherapy, as well as patients with SAD,[22] which, of course, is linked with improved cognition and memory.

A unique and important point about the Kent et al.[5] study mentioned earlier is that NASA satellite data were used to obtain natural sunlight exposure in the participants, whereas most existing studies are with artificial light sources.

Finally, this new finding that weather may affect cognition, as well as mood, has important clinical implications. It suggests that sunlight exposure has an independent relationship with cognition and depression, and that light therapy used in SAD may improve cognition, as well as mood. Hopefully future studies will continue to shed light, *every* pun intended, on these interesting clinical issues for us and our patients.

REFERENCES

1. Keller MC, Fredrickson BL, Ybarra O, et al. A warm heart and a clear head. The contingent effects of weather on mood and cognition. *Psychol Sci.* 2005;16(9):724-731.
2. Rosenthal NE, Sack DA, Gillin JC, et al. Seasonal affective disorder. A description of the syndrome and preliminary findings with light therapy. *Arch Gen Psychiatry.* 1984;41(1):72-80.
3. Van Someren EJ, Riemersma-Van Der Lek RF. Live to the rhythm, slave to the rhythm. *Sleep Med Rev.* 2007;11(6):465-484.
4. Howard VJ, Cushman M, Pulley L, et al. The reasons for geographic and racial differences in stroke study: objectives and design. *Neuroepidemiology.* 2005;25(3):135-143.
5. Kent ST, McClure LA, Crosson WL, et al. Effect of sunlight exposure on cognitive function among depressed and non-depressed participants: a REGARDS cross-sectional study. *Environ Health.* 2009;8:34.
6. Winkler D, Pjrek E, Iwaki R, Kasper S. Treatment of seasonal affective disorder. *Expert Rev Neurother.* 2006;6(7):1039-1048.
7. McColl SL, Veitch JA. Full-spectrum fluorescent lighting: a review of its effects on physiology and health. *Psychol Med.* 2001;31(6):949-964.

8. Srinivasan V, Smits M, Spence W, et al. Melatonin in mood disorders. *World J Biol Psychiatry.* 2006;7(3):138-151.
9. Lambert G, Reid C, Kaye D, Jennings G, Esler M. Increased suicide rate in the middle-aged and its association with hours of sunlight. *Am J Psychiatry.* 2003;160(4):793-795.
10. Miller AL. Epidemiology, etiology, and natural treatment of seasonal affective disorder. *Altern Med Rev.* 2005;10(1):5-13.
11. Leonard BE, Myint A. Changes in the immune system in depression and dementia: casual or coincidental effects: *Dialogues Clin Neurosci.* 2006;8(2):163-174.
12. Espiritu RC, Kripke DF, Ancoli-Israel S, et al. Low illumination experienced by San Diego adults: association with atypical depressive symptoms. *Biol Psychiatry.* 1994;35(6):403-407.
13. Haynes PL, Ancoli-Israel S, McQuaid J. Illuminating the impact of habitual behaviors in depression. *Chronobiol Int.* 2005;22(2):279-297.
14. Turner PL, Mainster MA. Circadian photoreception: ageing and the eye's important role in systemic health. *Br J Ophthalmol.* 2008;92(11):1439-1444.
15. Walker MP, Stickgold R. Sleep-dependent learning and memory consolidation. *Neuron.* 2004;44(1):121-133.
16. Khait VD, Huang YY, Malone KM, et al. Is there circannual variation of human platelet 5-HT(2A) binding in depression? *J Affect Disord.* 2002;71(1-3):249-258.
17. Srinivasan V, Pandi-Perumal SR, Cardinali DP, Poeggeler B, Hardeland R. Melatonin in Alzheimer's disease and other neurodegenerative disorders. *Behav Brain Funct.* 2006;2:15.
18. Jakovljevic M, Muck-Seler D, Pivac N, et al. Seasonal influence on platelet 5-HT levels in patients with recurrent major depression and schizophrenia. *Biol Psychiatry.* 1997;41(10):1028-1034.
19. Leppamaki S, Partonen T, Vakkuri O, et al. Effect of controlled-release melatonin on sleep quality, mood, and quality of life in subjects with seasonal or weather-associated changes in mood and behaviour. *Eur Neuropsychopharmacol.* 2003;13(3):137-145.
20. Golden RN, Gaynes BN, Ekstrom RD, et al. The efficacy of light therapy in the treatment of mood disorders: a review and meta-analysis of the evidence. *Am J Psychiatry.* 2005;162(4):656-662.
21. Dani C, Bertini G, Martelli E, et al. Effects of phototherapy on cerebral haemodynamics in preterm infants: is fibre-optic different from conventional phototherapy? *Dev Med Child Neurol.* 2004;46(2):114-118.
22. Matthew E, Vasile RG, Sachs G, et al. Regional cerebral blood flow changes after light therapy in seasonal affective disorder. *Nucl Med Commun.* 1996;17(6):475-479.

Role of Leptin in Depression and Obesity

QUESTION: "You mentioned that leptin may have a potential role in the treatment of depression. I've never heard of that; could you elaborate on the notion that there is a link between leptin, mood disorders, and obesity?"

Jon W. Draud, MS, MD:

This is an excellent question, and since its discovery approximately 10 years ago, leptin has been noted to be a critical mediator of energy homeostasis and serves as an adiposity negative feedback signal. There is also a putative role for leptin in the treatment of depression.

We know that depression is the most life-altering and prevalent of all mental disorders with a prevalence rate of about 20% worldwide. Current treatments for depression are all focused on compounds that exert therapeutic effects via promoting monoaminergic neurotransmission, but we know that these compounds often do not allow us to bring patients to a state of remission.[1,2]

Leptin is a peptide hormone secreted from adipocytes initially identified as an anti-obesity hormone. Newer evidence expands the potential role from energy homeostasis to regulation of reproduction and cognition.[3,4] Support for this expanded role is that leptin receptors are found in numerous brain regions, including the cortex, amygdala, and hippocampus—areas known to control emotion and mood.

In animal studies, rats exposed to chronic, but not acute stress showed decreased levels of plasma leptin.[5] Based on this, it was hypothesized that leptin insufficiency may contribute to depression-like behaviors, i.e., reduction of sucrose preference, which is seen as anhedonia in animal studies of depression.[6,7] Studies have shown that systemic administration of leptin can reverse this stress-induced reduction for sucrose preference.[5] Despair is another depressive symptom that can be measured by the forced Swim test and tail suspension test in studies, and on both of these measures the systemic administration of leptin was shown to produce a dose-dependent reduction of immobility, i.e., reduction of depressive symptoms.[5,8]

Human studies regarding leptin are limited, but there seems to be a loose association between reduced leptin levels and depression.[9-12] Interestingly, there is a 20% more likely incidence of depression in obese patients, and they actually have high leptin levels, but it is due to leptin resistance much like insulin resistance in diabetes. Therefore, leptin resistance seems to be the link to greater depression in obese patients.

Briefly, we will discuss the role of leptin as it relates to monoamines, HPA, and neurotrophins. Some studies show that serotonin content and metabolism are increased by leptin in the forebrain,[13,14] and others show that leptin enhances mesolimlic dopamine activity.[15] Accumulating evidence shows that leptin modulates HPA activity, which is implicated in depression. Chronic administration of leptin can reverse hypercortisolemia even prior to weight loss in mice,[16,17] and there is an inverse relationship between plasma leptin glucocorticoids and circadian rhythm activity.[18]

Finally, several studies link leptin to the neurotropic hypothesis of depression, and leptin actually has neurotropic effects itself. First, leptin deficiency leads to reduced brain volume in mice,[19,20] and leptin treatment causes protein synthesis and synaptic connectivity in rats.[21] Leptin has also been shown to be critical for certain pathway formations at hippocampus.[22,23]

In conclusion, there seems to be emerging evidence that leptin does have a role in possibly the etiology and future treatment of depressive disorders. The leptin hypothesis is complimentary to the other major prevailing hypotheses in depression (monoamine, HPA, and neurotrophic) and will be interesting to follow as clinicians.

REFERENCES

1. Berton O, Nestler EJ. New approaches to antidepressant drug discovery: beyond monaamines. *Nat Rev Neurosci.* 2006;7(2):137-151.
2. Frazer A. Pharmacology of antidepressants. *J Clin Psychopharmacol.* 1997;17(suppl 1):2S-18S.
3. Chehab FF. Leptin as a regulator of adipose mass and reproduction. *Trends Pharmacol Sci.* 2000;21(8):309-314.
4. Farr SA, Banks WA, Morley JE. Effects of leptin on memory processing. *Peptides.* 2006;27(6):1420-1425.
5. Lu XY, Kim CS, Frazer A. Zhang W. Leptin: a potential novel antidepressant. *Proc Natl Acad Sci U S A.* 2006;103(5):1593-1598.
6. Katz RJ. Animal model of depression: pharmacological sensitivity of a hedonic deficit. *Pharmacol Biochem Behav.* 1982;16(6):965-968.
7. Willner P. Chronic mild stress (CMS) revisited: consistency and behavioural-neurobiological cordance in the effects of CMS. *Neuropsychobiology.* 2005;52(2):90-110.
8. Kim CS, Huang TY, Garza J, et al. Leptin induces antidepressant-like behavioral effects and activates specific signal transduction pathways in the hippocampus and amygdala of mice. *Neuropsychopharmacology.* 2006;31(suppl 1S):S237-S238.
9. Jow GM, Yang TT, Chen CL. Leptin and cholesterol levels are low in major depressive disorder, but high in schizophrenia. *J Affect Disord.* 2006;90(1):21-27.
10. Kraus T, Haack M, Schuld A, Hinze-Selch D, Pollmacher T. Low leptin levels but normal body mass indices in patients with depression or schizophrenia. *Neuroendocrinology.* 2001;73(4):243-247.
11. Atmaca M, Kulogla M, Tezcan E, et al. Serum leptin and cholesterol values in suicide attempters. *Neuropsychobiology.* 2002;45(3):124-127.
12. Westling S, Ahren B, Traskman-Bendz L, Westrin A. Low CSF leptin in female suicide attempters with major depression. *J Affect Disord.* 2004;81(1):41-48.
13. Calapai G, Corica F, Corsonello A, et al. Leptin increases serotonin turnover by inhibition of brain nitric oxide synthesis. *J Clin Invest.* 1999;104(7):975-982.
14. Hastings JA, Wiesner G, Lambert G, et al. Influence of leptin on neurotransmitter overflow from the rat brain in vitro. *Regul Pept.* 2002;103(2-3):67-74.
15. Fulton S, Pissios P, Manchon RP, et al. Leptin regulation of the mesoaccumbens dopamine pathway. *Neuron.* 2006;51(6):811-822.
16. Chen H, Carlat O, Tartaglia LA, et al. Evidence that the diabetes gene encodes the leptin receptor: identification of a mutation in the leptin receptor gene in db/db mice. *Cell.* 1996;84(3):491-495.
17. Chua SC Jr, Chung WK, Wu-Peng XS, et al. Phenotypes of mouse diabetes and rat fatty due to mutations in the OB (leptin) receptor. *Science.* 1996;271(5251):994-996.

18. Stephens TW, Basinski M, Bristow PK, et al. The role of neuropeptide Y in the antiobesity action of the obese gene product. *Nature*. 1995;377(6549):530-532.
19. Licinio J, Mantzoros C, Negrao AB, et al. Human leptin levels are pulsatile and inversely related to pituitary-adrenal function. *Nat Med*. 1997;3(5):575-579.
20. Ahima RS, Bjorbaek C, Osei S, Flier JS. Regulation of neuronal and glial proteins by leptin: implications for brain development. *Endocrinology*. 1999;140(6):2755-2762.
21. Steppan CM, Swick AG. A role for leptin in brain development. *Biochem Biophys Res Commun*. 1999;256(3):600-602.
22. Proulx K, Clavel S, Nault G, Richard D, Walker CD. High neonatal leptin exposure enhances brain GR expression and feedback efficacy on the adrenocortical axis of developing rats. *Endocrinology*. 2001;142(11):4607-4616.
23. Bouret SG, Draper SJ, Simerly RB. Trophic action of leptin on hypothalamic neurons that regulate feeding. *Science*. 2004;304(5667):108-110.

Folate and Depression

QUESTION: **"I have been reading a lot about folate and folic acid in the treatment of depression. This does not make sense to me—isn't folate a vitamin? How can a vitamin play any role in the treatment of depression?"**

Rakesh Jain, MD, MPH:

Yes, folate and folic acid are indeed vitamins. Surprisingly, they potentially play a rather large role in the pathogenesis of depression! I understand your surprise; I really do. Digging into the literature on this topic has revealed many surprises that are worthy of further explorations. Yes, a "mere vitamin" may actually play an important role in depression. Let's look into this in greater detail, shall we?

By definition, a vitamin is a substance that is essential to human well-being, but it's not produced by the body and must be ingested. Folate is a water soluble vitamin that is found naturally in multiple foods. Folic acid is not a natural form of folate and must be converted by the human body to a usable form of folate. Folate has to be converted to L-methylfolate before it crosses the blood-brain barrier and penetrates the central nervous system.

There is emerging evidence, from epidemiological studies, that low consumption of folate and a lower blood level of folate increase the risk of suffering from major depression.[1-4] There is growing evidence that folate deficiency in pregnant mothers can adversely impact their babies.[2,5,6] There is also a body of literature that points to a relationship between low folate levels and cognitive decline.[7,8]

What role does folate play in depression? Well, if you think about it, it must play a pretty major role as it is intimately involved in the modulation of all three monoamines that play a central role in mood disorders—that being serotonin, norepinephrine, and dopamine.[9-12] It is a cofactor required in the optimum functioning of the rate limiting enzymatic steps needed to create the three neurotransmitters mentioned above. Do you see my point now? A mere vitamin can actually play a very significant role in depression!

At this point, you might be asking yourself this: If folate plays a role in the modulation of these three mood centric neurotransmitters, then does it have a role in treatment of depression? This question has not escaped the attention of several researchers.[13-15] Emerging evidence reveals that folate may actually have psychotropic properties, particularly in combination with antidepressants.

It's also important to note that folate may play an important role in physical health as well.[16] You probably have been keeping up with the literature on higher homocysteine blood levels and adverse outcomes.[17,18] There is modest evidence that folate may play a role in modulating homocysteine levels.[1,19]

I would say the following: As we move towards a better molecular understanding of depression and its treatment, we are realizing that important neurotransmitters in mood regulation (serotonin, norepinephrine, dopamine) have enzymatic modulators. Substances, such as folate, that regulate these enzymes may play a role in depression. Epidemiological, animal, human observational, and clinical studies all point to folate being one of the many factors involved in mood regulation.[20-23]

In conclusion, keep your eyes on the "folate story." We, of course, need more studies to fully understand this issue, and I encourage you (as I will be too!) to keep your eyes on emerging literature in this very interesting field of depression treatment. As the title of one recent article states, "Folate and Depression – a Neglected Problem,"[24] this issue has not been discussed very much in our field. I am glad you, by asking this question, have started a dialogue on a much ignored topic in depression care.

REFERENCES

1. Beydoun MA, Shroff MR, Beydoun HA, Zonderman AB. Serum folate, vitamin B-12, and homocysteine and their association with depressive symptoms among U.S. adults. *Psychosom Med*. 2010;[Epub ahead of print].

2. Van Dijk AE, Van Eijsden M, Stronks K, et al. Maternal depressive symptoms, serum folate status, and pregnancy outcome: results of the Amsterdam Born Children and their Development study. *Am J Obstet Gynecol*. 2010;[Epub ahead of print].

3. Williamson C. Dietary factors and depression in older people. *Br J Community Nurs*. 2009;14(10):422, 424-426.

4. Ng TP, Feng L, Niti M, et al. Folate, vitamin B12, homocysteine, and depressive symptoms in a population sample of older Chinese adults. *J Am Geriatr Soc*, 2009;57(5):871-876.

5. Devlin AM, Brain U, Austin J, Oberlander TF. Prenatal exposure to maternal depressed mood and the MTHFR C677T variant affect SLC6A4 methylation in infants at birth. *PLoS One*. 2010;5(8). pii: e12201.

6. Leung BM, Kaplan BJ. Perinatal depression: prevalence, risks, and the nutrition link--a review of the literature. *J Am Diet Assoc*. 2009;109(9):1566-1575.

7. Kronenberg G, Harms C, Sobol RW, et al. Folate deficiency induces neurodegeneration and brain dysfunction in mice lacking uracil DNA glycosylase. *J Neurosci*. 2008;28(28):7219-7230.

8. Aisen PS, Schneider LS, Sano M, et al. High-dose B vitamin supplementation and cognitive decline in Alzheimer disease: a randomized controlled trial. *JAMA*. 2008;300(5):1774-1783.

9. Fava M, Mischoulon D. Folate in depression: efficacy, safety, differences in formulations, and clinical issues. *J Clin Psychiatry*. 2009;70(Suppl 5):12-17.

10. Miller AL. The methylation, neurotransmitter, and antioxidant connections between folate and depression. *Altern Med Rev*. 2008;13(3):216-226.

11. Morris DW, Trivedi MH, Rush AJ. Folate and unipolar depression. *J Altern Complement Med*. 2008;14(3):277-285.

12. Brocardo PS, Budni J, Kaster MP, et al. Folic acid administration produces an antidepressant-like effect in mice: evidence for the involvement of the serotonergic and noradrenergic systems. *Neuropharmacology*. 2008;54(2):464-473.

13. Roberts SH, Bedson E, Hughes D, et al. Folate augmentation of treatment - evaluation for depression (FolATED): protocol of a randomised controlled trial. *BMC Psychiatry*. 2007;7:65.

14. Fava M. Augmenting antidepressants with folate: a clinical perspective. *J Clin Psychiatry*. 2007;68(Suppl 10):4-7.

15. Gariballa S, Forster S. Effects of dietary supplements on depressive symptoms in older patients: a randomised double-blind placebo-controlled trial. *Clin Nutr*. 2007;26(5):545-551.

16. Gopinath B, Flood VM, Rochtchina E, et al. Serum homocysteine and folate concentrations are associated with prevalent age-related hearing loss. *J Nutr*. 2010;140(8):1469-1474.

17. Almeida OP, McCaul K, Hankey GJ, et al. Homocysteine and depression in later life. *Arch Gen Psychiatry*. 2008;65(11):1286-1294.

18. Dimopoulos N, Piperi C, Salonicioti A, et al. Correlation of folate, vitamin B12 and homocysteine

plasma levels with depression in an elderly Greek population. *Clin Biochem.* 2007;40(9-10):604-608.

19. Bottiglieri T. Homocysteine and folate metabolism in depression. *Prog Neuropsychopharmacol Biol Psychiatry.* 2005;29(7):1103-1112.

20. Papakostas GI, Petersen T, Mischoulon D, et al. Serum folate, vitamin B12, and homocysteine in major depressive disorder, Part 2: predictors of relapse during the continuation phase of pharmacotherapy. *J Clin Psychiatry.* 2004;65(8):1096-1098.

21. Paul RT, McDonnell AP, Kelly CB. Folic acid: neurochemistry, metabolism and relationship to depression. *Hum Psychopharmacol.* 2004;19(7):477-488.

22. Murakami K, Miyake Y, Sasaki S, et al. Dietary Folate, Riboflavin, Vitamin B-6, and Vitamin B-12 and Depressive Symptoms in Early Adolescence: The Ryukyus Child Health Study. *Psychosom Med.* 2010;[Epub ahead of print].

23. Lazarou C, Kapsou M. The role of folic acid in prevention and treatment of depression: an overview of existing evidence and implications for practice. *Complement Ther Clin Pract.* 2010;16(3):161-166.

24. Young SN. Folate and depression--a neglected problem. *J Psychiatry Neurosci.* 2007;32(2):80-82.

SAMe and Folate

QUESTION: "I keep hearing about SAMe and folate as an 'add-on' treatment to standard antidepressant treatment. Does this make sense pharmacologically, and what is the evidence for their effectiveness?"

Rakesh Jain, MD, MPH:

You are right on many counts here. There has recently been a significant uptick in the conversation regarding SAMe and folate as "add-on" or augmentation therapies to suboptimum response to antidepressants. This conversation has been provoked by three facts: 1) we clinicians now have high quality, randomized studies with these two agents to examine for ourselves; 2) word of mouth regarding the effectiveness of these add-on agents is increasing clinician interest; and 3) the need for add-on therapy in depression care is so dire that clinicians' ears perk up anytime an option to help these unfortunate patients is being discussed.

But dire need alone cannot drive our decision to accept every "flavor of the month" augmentation therapy. We don't need fly-by-night options, popular one day and gone bust the next. We need well-studied and proven therapies. We need proof and scientific rationale for such therapies. So, let's examine the scientific rationale, then we will turn to clinical data.

Scientific Rationale

Let's return to our roots or to be more precise, let's go back to first-year medical school where we learned how neurotransmitters are "born." The neurotransmitters thought to play the biggest roles in depression—serotonin, norepinephrine, and dopamine—are all generated via pathways that start with amino acids and end with the neurotransmitters.[1,2] So far, so good, right? But hold on just a minute—how in the world is this process controlled and modulated? Are we all able to make exactly the same amounts of neurotransmitters? Here's where we learn further about the complexities of neurotransmitter generation.

Neurotransmitter genesis of all three of these neurotransmitters are controlled by enzymes that are often rate limiting, and they tightly control the rate of conversion of amino acids into neurotransmitters.[3-6] Let's also not forget that the activity of these enzymes is controlled by our genotype for that enzyme; some of us have good activity of these enzymes, and some of us don't.[3] Let's also remember there are multiple cofactors needed in this process. In other words, enzymes are not sufficient by themselves to create the neurotransmitter; cofactors play a central and critical role in creating these vitally needed neurotransmitters.[1]

What do these cofactors do?

These cofactors (SAMe and folate are cofactors) are considered to be "methyl donors."

This donation of a methyl group by these cofactors is needed before a neurotransmitter is generated. This donation of the methyl group (*methyl is CH_3*) is amazingly important in the *one carbon metabolism cycle* of neurotransmitter synthesis.[1,7]

I hope I haven't lost you in all this technical jibber-jabber! But this is important information for the modern-day clinician.

Let's summarize what we have learned so far:

– Neurotransmitters such as serotonin, norepinephrine, and dopamine are critical for mood regulation and depression to occur, in part because of impairment in these neurotransmitters' functioning.

– The pathway to neurotransmitter synthesis requires multiple things—not the least of them are enzymes and cofactors.

– Impairment in the functioning of these enzymes or cofactors will result in neurotransmitter generation impairment.

– SAMe and folate are important cofactors in neurotransmitter generation pathways.

To continue this fascinating story, let's find out a little more about the cofactors SAMe and folate. What are they? Where do they come from? SAMe stands for s-adenosylmethionine. Yep, quite a mouthful; hence it might be easier to just call it SAMe, right?! The parent of SAMe is the amino acid methionine. SAMe is famous for being perhaps the top methyl donor in the process that creates the neurotransmitters. Once SAMe donates its methyl group, it becomes homocysteine. Homocysteine, which if it accumulates can cause adverse health effects,[4,6,8,9] needs remethylation in order to become SAMe again – and here is where folate steps in.

Turning our attention to folate, let's remember that the active form of folate is 5-MTHF (5-methyltetrahydrofolate)—another mouthful of a word! So let's just call it MTHF or L-methylfolate. Dietary folate and supplemental folate need conversion into L-methylfolate before they can cross the blood brain barrier and participate in the neurotransmitter synthesis. This is a tricky issue, as genetic polymorphisms for the creation of L-methylfolate are unusually common (and appear to be even more common in individuals with major depression). There is a commercially available form of L-methylfolate, which means one can bypass all the various tricky enzymatic steps by taking the active form of folate. More on this later.

At least theoretically you can see what these two substances—SAMe and folate—are of such interest to those of us who take care of people who suffer from depression, right? But at the end of the day, we are less interested in these theories and more interested in finding out what happens when the "rubber meets the road"—that is, what do the clinical studies show?

Clinical Studies

SAMe has had a long and storied history in psychopharmacological research, but many older studies suffered from the challenge of small sample sizes and differing methodologies; however, the overall data suggests that SAMe is an effective agent.[10-16] Additionally, a recent, very well conducted study by Papakostas and colleagues has created quite a buzz.[17] This study showed SAMe to be an effective and well-tolerated add-on agent when a selective serotonin reuptake inhibitor (SSRI) alone was not fully effective. The response rates were double in the SAMe arm as compared to placebo. Impressive indeed.

In regards to folate, similar issues apply. Earlier studies dating back to 1990 and even earlier appear to show a pretty clear signal of benefit, but not until recently have we had the kind of evidence needed to convince us clinicians to give folate a second look.[2,18-21] Clinical studies over the last several decades have offered us intriguing information about folate as a potential antidepressant.[8,22-27] We now have two studies, conducted not with folic acid, which requires a large number of enzymatic changes before it becomes the active, blood-barrier crossing form of folate—L-methylfolate,[1] but with L-methylfolate itself. Ginsberg and colleagues demonstrated in an open-label, naturalized, single center study that L-methyfolate when added to SSRI or serotonin-norepinephrine reuptake inhibitors (SNRIs) at the beginning of therapy was more effective than only using an SSRI or SNRI.[28] Almost immediately after that, Papakostas and colleagues presented a poster at the European Congress of Psychiatry on an extremely well-conducted blinded, randomized study of L-methylfolate augmentation to SSRI nonresponders, showing a greater than two-fold increase in response rates.[29]

In response to your question, I will say this—the emerging basic science and clinical studies literature is supportive of considering SAMe and folate as viable antidepressant augmentation options. There is reason for caution too. We have a growing, but still limited database, and long-term studies for efficacy and safety are very limited. Excessive exuberance regarding these two options is not yet warranted. Certainly, we are in need of more studies, and I suspect we will see a number of them in the next few months to years. Keep your eyes peeled for them. The needs of our antidepressant-treated, but suboptimally responsive, patients are significant, and we welcome all effective options to the table.

REFERENCES

1. Miller AL. The methylation, neurotransmitter, and antioxidant connections between folate and depression. *Alt Med Rev*. 2008;13(3):216-226.
2. Abou-Saleh MT, Coppen A. The biology of folate in depression: implications for nutritional hypotheses of the psychoses. *J Psychiatr Res*. 1986;20(2):91-101.
3. Bjelland I, Tell GS, Vollset SE, Refsum M, Ueland PM. Folate, vitamin B12, homocysteine, and the MTHFR 677C->T polymorphism in anxiety and depression: the Hordaland Homocysteine Study. *Arch Gen Psychiatry*. 2003;60(6):618-626.
4. Bottiglieri T. Homocysteine and folate metabolism in depression. *Prog Neuropsychopharmacol Biol Psychiatry*. 2005;29(7):1103-1112.
5. Bottiglieri T, Hyland K, Laundy M, et al. Folate deficiency, biopterin and monoamine metabolism in depression. *Psychol Med*. 1992;22(4):871-876.
6. Bottiglieri T, Laundy M, Crellin R, et al. Homocysteine, folate, methylation, and monoamine metabolism in depression. *J Neurol Neurosurg Psychiatry*. 2000;69(2):228-232.
7. Morris DW, Trivedi MH, Rush AJ. Folate and unipolar depression. *J Altern Complement Med*.

2008;14(3):277-285.

8. Papakostas GI, Petersen T, Mischoulon D, et al. Serum folate, vitamin B12, and homocysteine in major depressive disorder, Part 1: predictors of clinical response in fluoxetine-resistant depression. *J Clin Psychiatry*. 2004;65(8):1090-1095.

9. Tiemeier H, van Tuijl HR, Hofman A, et al. Vitamin B12, folate, and homocysteine in depression: the Rotterdam Study. *Am J Psychiatry*. 2002;159(12):2099-2101.

10. Andreoli VM, Maffei F, Tonon GC. S-adenosyl-L-methionine (SAMe) blood levels in schizophrenia and depression. *Monogr Gesamtgeb Psychiatr Psychiatry Ser*. 1978;18:147-150.

11. Baime MJ. Review: SAMe reduces symptoms in depression, osteoarthritis, and liver disease. *ACP J Club*. 2003;139(1):20.

12. Genedani S, Saltini S, Benelli A, Filaferro M, Bertolini A. Influence of SAMe on the modifications of brain polyamine levels in an animal model of depression. *Neuroreport*. 2001;12(18):3939-3942.

13. Janicak PG, Lipinski J, Davis JM, Altman E, Sharma RP. Parenteral S-adenosyl-methionine (SAMe) in depression: literature review and preliminary data. *Psychopharmacol Bull*. 1989;25(2):238-242.

14. Ramos L. SAMe as a supplement: can it really help treat depression and arthritis? *J Am Diet Assoc*. 2000;100(4):414.

15. Williams AL, Girard C, Jui D, Sabina A, Katz DL. S-adenosylmethionine (SAMe) as treatment for depression: a systematic review. *Clin Invest Med*. 2005;28(3):132-139.

16. Young SN. Are SAMe and 5-HTP safe and effective treatments for depression? *J Psychiatry Neurosci*. 2003;28(6):471.

17. Papakostas GI, Mischoulon D, Shyu I, Alpert JE, Fava M. S-adenosyl methionine (SAMe) augmentation of serotonin reuptake inhibitors for antidepressant nonresponders with major depressive disorder: a double-blind, randomized clinical trial. *Am J Psychiatry*. 2010;167(8):942-948.

18. Abou-Saleh MT, Coppen A. Serum and red blood cell folate in depression. *Acta Psychiatr Scand*. 1989;80(1):78-82.

19. Alpert JE, Fava M. Nutrition and depression: the role of folate. *Nutr Rev*. 1997;55(5):145-149.

20. Alpert JE, Mischoulon D, Nierenberg AA, Fava M. Nutrition and depression: focus on folate. *Nutrition*. 2000;16(7-8):544-546.

21. Bjelland I, Ueland PM, Vollset SE. Folate and depression. *Psychother Psychosom*. 2003;72(2):59-60.

22. Fava M, Mischoulon D. Folate in depression: efficacy, safety, differences in formulations, and clinical issues. *J Clin Psychiatry*. 2009;70(Suppl 5):12-17.

23. Gilbody S, Lightfoot T, Sheldon T. Is low folate a risk factor for depression? A meta-analysis and exploration of heterogeneity. *J Epidemiol Community Health*. 2007;61(7):631-637.

24. Mischoulon D, Raab MF. The role of folate in depression and dementia. *J Clin Psychiatry*. 2007;68(Suppl 10):28-33.

25. Miyake Y, Sasaki S, Tanaka K, et al. Dietary folate and vitamins B12, B6, and B2 intake and the risk of postpartum depression in Japan: the Osaka Maternal and Child Health Study. *J Affect Disord*. 2006;96(1-2):133-138.

26. Morris MS, Fava M, Jacques PF, Selhub J, Rosenberg IH. Depression and folate status in the US Population. *Psychother Psychosom*. 2003;72(2):80-87.

27. Roberts SH, Bedson E, Hughes D, et al. Folate augmentation of treatment - evaluation for depression (FolATED): protocol of a randomised controlled trial. *BMC Psychiatry*. 2007;7:65.

28. Ginsberg LD, Oubre AY, Daoud YA. L-methylfolate plus SSRI or SNRI from treatment initiation compared to SSRI or SNRI monotherapy in a major depressive disorder. *Innov Clin Neurosci*. 2011;8(1):19-28.

29. Papakostas GI, Shelton RC, Zajecka J, et al. L-methylfolate as adjunctive therapy for selective serotonin reuptake inhibitor-resistant major depressive disorder: results of two randomized, double-blind, parallel-sequential trials. Poster presented at: European Congress of Psychiatry; March 14, 2011; Vienna, Austria.

Mindfulness-Based Cognitive Therapy

QUESTION: "I have been hearing a lot about mindfulness, meditation, and cognitive therapy being combined to help prevent relapses in depression. Tell me more about it."

Rakesh Jain, MD, MPH:

There is currently a virtual explosion in the knowledge base regarding this topic. Cognitive-behavioral therapy (CBT) is by now an established and efficacious intervention for many different psychiatric conditions. In the last decade, a modified version of CBT—modified to include elements of meditation derived from ancient Eastern practices—has been studied and now vividly demonstrates to be effective in depression. This hybrid form of therapy is called mindfulness-based cognitive therapy (MBCT), and I for one am entirely sold on it.

Let me lay out a scientific and clinical case for why all of us, regardless of our practice setting, should be aware of this new manual and experiential-based therapy, and offer it to our patients.

First, let's examine the shortcomings in our current depression armamentarium. Pharmacological treatment of depression is indeed making great progress. However, let's be truthful with each other, shall we—the rates of response, remission, and relapse (the curse of the three Rs as I call it) — remain scandalously high. If the truth be told, the Emperor is indeed naked, or at best, is partly clothed. An issue facing American psychiatry, and for that matter global psychiatry, is that we are overly reliant on medications as a path of salvation for our patients. CBT, physical exercise, and improved socialization are all proven non-pharmacological treatments in depression.

Before we take a look at MBCT techniques, let's examine the neurobiological signature of meditation. Considerable and replicated evidence shows that people who meditate on a regular basis are volumetrically different than non-meditators. This includes increased volumes of hippocampus even with as little as an eight-week course of meditation-based stress reduction,[1] to decreased volume of amygdala also after an eight-week similar course of practice.[2] But there is more: studies demonstrate that meditation also has a positive effect on the autonomic and inflammatory systems[3]—both as you well know, are deeply dysregulated in individuals suffering from major depression. Additionally, evidence points to meditation practice as being helpful in pain modulation,[4] this presumably occurring as a result of the activation of the pain inhibitory parts of our brains (the cingulate and the insular cortex).

How exactly does MBCT work? Some work has been done to examine the pathways by which this happens. MBCT may "turn down" an individual's cognitive reactivity,[5] a well known cause of both depression and its relapse. If practiced regularly, MBCT can break the cycle of depressive thinking.

Research and clinical evidence for MBCT's effectiveness is ever growing. We now have evidence for its effectiveness in generalized anxiety disorder,[6] panic disorder,[7] treatment-resistant depression,[8] and, most recently, in prevention of relapse in major depression after stabilization with medications and then discontinuation.[9]

This last study, published by Segal and colleagues, is truly impressive as MBCT was shown to be as effective in relapse prevention as continuation of pharmacotherapy. They have also published a manual for us clinicians: *Mindfulness-Based Cognitive Therapy for Depression: A New Approach to Preventing Relapse.* I would encourage you to read it, like I have, should you have an active interest in offering MBCT to your patients. Remember, MBCT can be offered to patients both on medication and not on them. Additionally, there is a patient, self-guided MBCT book also written by this same group that I have been recommending to my patients: *The Mindful Way Through Depression: Freeing Yourself from Chronic Unhappiness.* A big plus of this second book is that it includes an audio CD that patients can use for meditation practice.

Ancient mindful meditation wisdom when married to Western cognitive therapy principals produces a powerful new treatment modality called MBCT. I believe it's time for all of us to learn more about it, and apply it in our practices!

REFERENCES

1. Holzel BK, Carmody J, Vangel M, et al. Mindfulness practice leads to increases in regional brain gray matter density. *Psychiatry Res.* 2011;191(1):36-43.

2. Holzel BK, Carmody J, Evans KC, et al. Stress reduction correlates with structural changes in the amygdala. *Soc Cogn Affect Neurosci.* 2010;5(1):11-17.

3. Kiecolt-Glaser JK, Christian L, Preston H, et al. Stress, inflammation, and yoga practice. *Psychosom Med.* 2010;72(2):113-121.

4. Brown CA, Jones AK. Meditation experience predicts less negative appraisal of pain: electrophysiological evidence for the involvement of anticipatory neural responses. *Pain.* 2010;150(3):428-438.

5. Kuyken W, Watkins E, Holden E, et al. How does mindfulness-based cognitive therapy work? *Behav Res Ther.* 2010;48(11):1105-1112.

6. Evans S, Ferrando S, Findler M, et al. Mindfulness-based cognitive therapy for generalized anxiety disorder. *J Anxiety Disord.* 2008;22(4):716-721.

7. Kim B, Lee SH, Kim YH, et al. Effectiveness of a mindfulness-based cognitive therapy program as an adjunct to pharmacotherapy in patients with panic disorder. *J Anxiety Disord.* 2010;24(6):590-595.

8. Kenny MA, Williams JM. Treatment-resistant depressed patients show a good response to Mindfulness-based Cognitive Therapy. *Behav Res Ther.* 2007;45(3):617-625.

9. Segal ZV, Bieling P, Young T, et al. Antidepressant monotherapy vs sequential pharmacotherapy and mindfulness-based cognitive therapy, or placebo, for relapse prophylaxis in recurrent depression. *Arch Gen Psychiatry.* 2010;67(12):1256-1264.

Integrative Approaches to Treatment-Resistant Depression

QUESTION: "Is it ever appropriate for me to tell my treatment-refractory patients, 'There's nothing more that can be done to help you,' that, unfortunately, there is no further hope of helping them?"

Rakesh Jain, MD, MPH:

Let me respond by telling a recent, personal story. My sister-in-law was diagnosed with lung cancer two years ago and, despite initial success in treatment, the cancer came back aggressively. She was taken care of by one of the finest oncology teams anywhere in the United States. Multiple treatments were tried, alas, no success. Her health deteriorated remarkably, and her quality of life fell sharply.

We were asked by the doctors to consider stopping treatment and offered us hospice care. They said, realistically speaking, my sister-in-law's chances of survival beyond four weeks were less than 1%. We were told her condition was treatment refractory, and they had no more to offer.

By this time, my sister-in-law was in a coma, and the family turned to me (as the only physician in the family) and asked for my opinion. I told them that, honestly, there was no realistic hope of recovery. They did decide to stop treatment, turned to hospice care, and six days later my sister-in-law died peacefully. This happened about six months ago.

I am at peace in my heart that I gave the right advice. The situation was hopeless and further treatment was simply cruel and unproductive. Now, I share this very personal story with all of you to say that there are circumstances in clinical medicine where making a reasoned judgment to withhold any further treatment is prudent and humane.

However, in the treatment of depression, this is not—emphatically *not*—the way to go. I want to be very clear on this point. I wish to state as clearly as I can: in the treatment of depression, even in the refractory patients, there is never a time to recommend withholding treatment or from not attempting further treatment trials.

You have the right to question my stance. You may be asking yourself, "Is he just being a wild-eyed optimist or is his thinking based on good science?" This is a fair question. Let me present some evidence that supports my position of never giving up on any patient afflicted with depression, no matter how refractory it seems at this point.

First of all, let's examine evidence from one of our premier studies in depression—the famed STAR*D study.[1,2] If you recall, more and more patients kept achieving remission as patients moved from one step to another. Certainly, the rates kept going lower with each step, but note this carefully, never did a step lead to zero increase in gain. Each step produced incremental benefit, no matter how small it was. This is evidence that therapeutic nihilism has no place in the treatment of depression.

We now have FDA options approved specifically for treatment refractory depression and for suboptimally treated depression.[3-5] Thyroid augmentation is continuing to show promise.[6] The number of options is increasing rapidly. We clinicians have more tools at our disposal today than we have ever had.

Let's not forget that well-controlled studies of psychotherapy in depression reveal the power of these interventions.[7] Happily, it's one more option to help our patients with treatment-resistant depression. Even less reason to practice therapeutic negativity.

What about the multiple somatic treatments available to us? Electroconvulsive therapy is still one of great friends for treatment refractory patients, and I feel more patients should be offered this as a treatment option when they run into treatment refractoriness (both unipolar and bipolar depression).[8] The advent of vagus nerve stimulation[9] and transcranial magnetic stimulation[10] for difficult-to-treat depression are welcome additions to our weaponry. Deep brain stimulation[11,12] is showing promising results in this population. Even psychosurgery for extraordinarily refractory patients shows promise.[13]

This Q&A is not to discuss a step-by-step approach to treating refractory patients afflicted with depression, but rather to vigorously defend the position that it's *never* appropriate to give up hope. Giving up hope is not appropriate for the patient or the clinician who take care of them. This is not a "pie in the sky" kind of approach. It's scenically, ethically, and realistically an accurate position for all to take. There is always hope for even the most treatment refractory depressed patient out there. I believe this personally, and I believe science backs up this position.

REFERENCES

1. Warden D, Rush AJ, Trivedi MH, et al. The STAR*D Project results: a comprehensive review of findings. *Curr Psychiatry Rep.* 2007;9(6):449-459.
2. Rush AJ. STAR*D: what have we learned? *Am J Psychiatry.* 2007;164(2):201-204.
3. Bobo WV, Shelton RC. Efficacy, safety and tolerability of Symbyax for acute-phase management of treatment-resistant depression. *Expert Rev Neurother.* 2010;10(5):651-670.
4. Berman RM, Fava M, Thase ME, et al. Aripiprazole augmentation in major depressive disorder: a double-blind, placebo-controlled study in patients with inadequate response to antidepressants. *CNS Spectr.* 2009;14(4):197-206.
5. Bauer M, Pretorius HW, Constant EL, et al. Extended-release quetiapine as adjunct to an antidepressant in patients with major depressive disorder: results of a randomized, placebo-controlled, double-blind study. *J Clin Psychiatry.* 2009;70(4):540-549.
6. Kelly TF, Lieberman DZ. Long term augmentation with T3 in refractory major depression. *J Affect Disord.* 2009;115(1-2):230-233.
7. Matsunaga M, Okamoto Y, Suzuki S, et al. Psychosocial functioning in patients with Treatment-Resistant Depression after group cognitive behavioral therapy. *BMC Psychiatry.* 2010;10:22.
8. Medda P, Perugi G, Zanello S, et al. Comparative response to electroconvulsive therapy in medication-resistant bipolar I patients with depression and mixed state. *J ECT.* 2010;26(2):82-86.
9. Ansari S, Chaudhri K, Al Moutaery KA. Vagus nerve stimulation: indications and limitations. *Acta Neurochir Suppl.* 2007;97(pt 2):281-286.

10. Krisanaprakornkit T, Paholpak S, Tassaniyom K, Pimpanit V. Transcranial magnetic stimulation for treatment resistant depression: six case reports and review. *J Med Assoc Thai.* 2010;93(5):580-586.

11. Mohr P. Deep brain stimulation in psychiatry. *Neuro Endocrinol Lett.* 2008;29(suppl 1):123-132.

12. Pereira EA, Green AL, Nandi D, Aziz TZ. Deep brain stimulation: indications and evidence. *Expert Rev Med Devices.* 2007;4(5):591-603.

13. Steele JD, Christmas D, Eljamel MS, Matthews K. Anterior cingulotomy for major depression: clinical outcome and relationship to lesion characteristics. *Biol Psychiatry.* 2008;63(7):670-677.

Chapter 5

THOUGHT AND MOOD DISORDERS CONTINUUM

Thought and Mood Disorders Continuum

QUESTION: "Please comment on the history of the dichotomy between schizophrenia and bipolar disorders."

Jon W. Draud, MS, MD:

This will be a brief posting that will begin to answer the above question, and will be expounded seeing as there are so many aspects to be explored. The distinction between so called "thought and mood disorders" dates to the late 1800s and is otherwise known as the Kraepelinian dichotomy. Emil Kraepelin established this categorical division in 1880, but interestingly recanted his own thinking in a book published in 1920—six years before his death.

I happen to fall into the camp who believes there is no real clear-cut division, and that thought and mood disorders are better capitalized along a continuum. As mentioned, we will explore this continuum concept in detail over the coming months, but for now will mention a few thoughts on the scientific basis for establishing a bonafide psychiatric disease state. In a recent paper, Lake lists six criteria that must be met to establish the existence of psychiatric diseases, given that there are no discreet pathophysiological tests that are diagnostic.[1] The criteria are: 1) symptoms that are clearly unique to one disease; 2) consistent epidemiology; 3) consistent response to medications; 4) generally consistent course and outcome; 5) an increased heritability in first-degree relatives; and 6) the identification of specific genetic susceptibility loci.

Lake hypothesizes, and I generally agree, that schizophrenia is better thought of as a psychotic mood disorder, and feels that bipolar disorder (BD) meets the six criteria where schizophrenia does not.

Regarding the first criterion, the signs and symptoms of classic BD are quite unique and have been recognized for over 2,000 years. There is a subset of psychotic and unremitting patients with BD that, over time, resemble patients classically diagnosed with schizophrenia. There is clear overlap epidemiologically between BD and schizophrenia as reviewed by Berettini.[2]

Regarding the third criterion, lithium and other mood stabilizing agents generally reduce cycling in BD, and traditional antidepressants induce switching to mania or hypomania 15% of the time. Antipsychotics are, on the other hand, effective in both diagnostic types of patients providing no clarity. Then regarding cycling, though the length is variable, there tends to be a consistent decrease in cycle length with each episode of bipolarity. Psychotic symptoms are considered disease non-specific, though many tend to jump to a schizophrenia bias diagnostically when present.

Finally, genetically, there is mounting evidence that BD is clinically distinct, whereas the majority of evidence shows that BD and schizophrenia do not "breed true" and seems to overlap tremendously.

This is a controversial topic that we will continue to explore. In my opinion, this continuum concept is a critical one for our field and has ultimately tremendous clinical and practical implications.

REFERENCES

1. Lake CR. The validity of schizophrenia vs. bipolar disorder. *Psychiatric Annals*. 2010;40(2):77-87.
2. Berrettini WH. Are schizophrenic and bipolar disorders related? A review of family and molecular studies. *Biol Psychiatry*. 2000;48(6):531-538.

Bipolar Spectrum Disorders in the *Diagnostic and Statistical Manual of Mental Disorders-V*

QUESTION: "What will be the representation of the Bipolar Spectrum Disorders in the *Diagnostic and Statistical Manual of Mental Disorders-V* (*DSM-V*)?"

Rakesh Jain, MD, MPH:

There is no doubt that the single most discussed, argued over, and controversial topic is what you are alluding to—What will *DSM-V* do with the Bipolar Spectrum Disorders!

Why this controversy? The reason is simply: we clinicians are seeing a very significant number of patients who clearly have mood symptoms that do not fit either major depression, nor *DSM-IV*-defined Bipolar I or II Disorders. These patients also often do poorly on antidepressants. So what do we call them? A search of *DSM-IV* leaves many of these patients without a "diagnostic home." This is not just an academic matter where we clinicians feel compelled to label patients correctly—the diagnosis we give our patients often has profound short- and long-term implications. An error can have significant negative implications, such as incorrect medication choices, treatment misadventures, loss of patient confidence in the psychiatric profession, and worse.

Therefore, we are often forced to use terminology such as "Bipolar Spectrum Disorder" to label these patients who have some symptoms from the mood disorder criteria, but not enough to be fully inclusive. What is not in doubt is that these patients are suffering from their symptoms. The problem is that *DSM-IV* is completely silent on the spectrum issue: each clinician creates their own definition of what is a spectrum and what isn't. Speaking for myself, my acceptance of the spectrum concept of bipolar disorder has lead to significantly better treatment outcomes for many of my patients. My treatment choices are better and more effective now that I am willing to accept that many patients will not neatly fit any categories, but I still have an obligation to help them.

Let's quickly examine a recent article by Angst and colleagues.[1] These data are from the National Comorbidity Survey Replication study (NCS-R), which finds a whopping 40% of patients with major depression have subthreshold hypomanic symptoms. An amazing 40%! This is not, therefore, a rare event. What would we call these patients—bipolar? Well, we can't if we stick to *DSM-IV* criteria, so we end up using the amorphous phrase: Bipolar Spectrum Disorder.

This categorical/dimensional split is vexing to both clinicians and researchers. Vieta and Phillips, in a recent article, have tackled this topic head on, and I recommend reading their article.[2]

DSM-V, expected to come to life in the next few years, has indeed taken an interest in this issue. While the American Psychiatric Association (APA) is at the point of gathering feedback, it has put out some suggested criteria. While one cannot predict what the ultimate shape of *DSM-V* will be in regards to this issue, one thing appears to be clear—it will have a more dimensional approach to diagnosis, in contrast to just a categorical approach. I see both advantages and disadvantages to this changed approach, but mostly advantages.

The advantages: the dimensional approach will be a far better way to diagnose nearly all patients we see in our practices. For example, new research studies will look at treatment outcomes in dimensionally ill patients, and not just the categorically defined patients; and patients with both mild and severe illnesses will justifiably be given psychiatric attention. The downside is the backlash one can expect from the lay public and the press. They might raise objections such as: Is Psychiatry trying to say everyone has mental illness? If everyone has some symptoms, does it mean everyone is ill, and therefore should take medications? Is the APA trying to be a marketing tool for pharmaceutical companies in order to sell more medications? While these points are false and without merit, we mental health clinicians will have to deal with these questions if and when the dimensional approach to making a diagnosis becomes part of *DSM-V*.

If you wish to read more on this issue straight from the *DSM-V* committee, check out this link: www.dsm5.org/ProposedRevisions/Pages/MoodDisorders.aspx.

REFERENCES
1. Angst J, Cui L, Swendsen J, et al. Major depressive disorder with subthreshold bipolarity in the National Comorbidity Survey Replication. *Am J Psychiatry.* 2010;[Epub ahead of print].
2. Vieta E, Phillips ML. Deconstructing bipolar disorder: a critical review of its diagnostic validity and a proposal for DSM-V and ICD-11. *Schizophr Bull.* 2007;33(4):886-892.

Mixed Depression

QUESTION: "Please discuss the concept termed 'mixed depression.'"

Jon W. Draud, MS, MD:

Many feel that "mixed states," which implies a patient suffering with opposite polarity symptoms within the same mood episode, is the bridge between the artificial divisions between unipolar depression and bipolar depression. The artificial dichotomy between unipolar states and bipolar states has fallen under much scrutiny of late, and terms like "agitated depression" and "irritable depression" or mixed depressions may be better described as patients along a "bipolar spectrum."

Mixed depression has been defined as a combination of depression and three or more intradepressive hypomanic symptoms. Mood disorders have classically been categorically split into bipolar disorders and unipolar disorders. This division is being questioned by the concepts of mood disorder continuum or spectrum.

Benazzi has recently reviewed these concepts.[1,2] Benazzi also assessed the distribution of intradepressive hypomanic symptoms between major depressive disorder (MDD) and bipolar II disorder (BP-II), as well as examined a potential dose-response relationship between bipolar family history and intradepressive hypomanic symptoms.[3]

Patients were interviewed by an experienced clinician with 21 years of practice experience in an outpatient setting. A total of 389 BP-II and 261 MDD outpatients were included, free of substance abuse, borderline personality disorders, or significant medical, cognitive, or substance abuse issues.

The distribution of intradepressive hypomanic symptoms between BP-II and MDD was not bi-modal. Bipolar II depression did seem to have more recurrences, a stronger family history of bipolarity, and a lower age of onset plus a greater overall number of intradepressive hypomanic symptoms compared to MDD, but there was no true bi-modality established. A dose-response relationship was found between intradepressive hypomanic symptoms and bipolar family history loading. Benazzi concluded that these findings question the categorical division of BP-II and MDD, and may support the spectrum view of mood disorders.

REFERENCES
1. Benazzi F. Mood patterns and classification in bipolar disorder. *Curr Opin Psychiatry*. 2006;19(1):1-8.
2. Benazzi F. The relationship of major depressive disorder to bipolar disorder: continuous or discontinuous? *Curr Psychiatry Rep*. 2005;7(6):462-470.
3. Benazzi F. The continuum/spectrum concept of mood disorders: is mixed depression the basic link? *Eur Arch Psychiatry Clin Neurosci*. 2006;256(8):512-515.

Pseudounipolar Depression

QUESTION: "I have recently heard a lecture about 'pseudounipolar' depression. Does this form of mood disorder really exist?"

Vladimir Maletic, MS, MD:

Unfortunately, there is a lack of consensus about the existence of "pseudounipolar" depression. Many patients who are diagnosed as depressive disorder NOS or treatment-resistant depression display a combination of depressive symptomatology combined with two or more hypomanic/manic symptoms, yet they do not meet syndromal criteria for any other mood state. Most frequently patients will complain of depression, social anxiety, obsessive tendencies, irritability, emotional lability, "crowded mind," and difficulty falling asleep because their mind "will just not turn off."

Our diagnostic taxonomy offers little help; unipolar and bipolar depression have the same criteria. Therefore, one must rely on information about mania or hypomania to make the distinction. Patients will seldom spontaneously report hypomanic symptoms: sometimes it is due to lack of awareness; at other times, it is reluctance to discuss embarrassing behaviors from the past.

Using a structured interview, Cassano and colleagues[1] discovered frequent presence of hypomanic symptoms in context of unipolar depression. Hypomanic symptoms were not normally distributed; about one-third of the patients with depression accounted for most of the hypomanic/manic symptoms. These patients were, for the research purposes, labeled as "pseudounipolar."[2] Described depressive variant is characterized by presence of a few hypomanic symptoms and more pronounced social anxiety, panic attacks, and obsessive tendencies relative to other patients suffering from depression.[2] Proper recognition of "pseudounipolar" depression may be of significant clinical relevance since these patients are less likely to respond to conventional antidepressant treatments and more likely to have psychotic features.[3] They will often benefit from adjunct mood-stabilizing agents.

REFERENCES
1. Cassano GB, Rucci P, Frank E, et al. The mood spectrum in unipolar and bipolar disorder: arguments for a unitary approach. *Am J Psychiatry*. 2004;161(7):1264-1269.
2. Cassano GB. Threshold and subthreshold mania in mood and anxiety disorders. Sixth International Conference on Bipolar Disorder; June 16-18, 2005; Pittsburgh, PA.
3. Smith DJ, Forty L, Russell E, et al. Sub-threshold manic symptoms in recurrent major depressive disorder are a marker for poor outcome. *Acta Psychiatr Scand*. 2009;119(4):325-329.

Organic Depression

QUESTION: "How much of what was presented today (re: organic depression) would hold for reactive (situational) depression? For example, a man in his 50s with no history of notable depression who has lost his job with two children in college and becomes significantly depressed for the first time?"

Charles Raison, MD:

This is a great question that takes us directly to the role played by a person's physiology versus environment in the onset of depression. Let me get my theoretical biases right out in front of this community forum. Short of depression after a stroke or something similar, I do not believe that "organic" depression exists, or if it does, it is very rare. This does not mean that genes don't contribute to depression or that depression isn't a biological disorder, only that, when it comes to depression, the person and the environment are like a lock and key not easily separated. Note that my colleagues and I have somewhat different views of this matter. I'm purposely being a little provocative in hopes that Dr. Rakesh Jain will take up the gene cause in a response.

Let me elaborate. The general consensus of our field is that major depression is mostly an environmental condition.[1] But it is complicated.

First, the role of the environment gets stronger and stronger the more closely one looks at environment. For example Kenneth Kendler—probably our field's leader in these matters—has shown that as one moves from a general family environment to the particular micro-environment around each child, the role of environment grows proportionately.[2] Some kids fit better with their parents than others, and these sorts of very personal environmental factors turn out to be powerful in terms of setting up a person's physiology for depression.

Second, Kendler has also shown that people's genes also seem to contribute to what type of environments they select themselves into. Genes that increase the risk for depression also seem to drive people toward environments likely to be depressogenic.[1,3,4] Interestingly, the opposite appears to be true at the level of whole societies. It turns out that societies with a very high prevalence of the short form of the serotonin transporter polymorphism (repeatedly shown to increase the risk of depression in response to stress) also evolve cultural patterns—such as collectivism—that protect against depression, with the result that depression prevalence is lower in these groups than in populations (such as the United States) in which the prevalence of the short form of the serotonin polymorphism is much lower.[5]

So, if I were to simplify the situation between genes and environment in the development of depression, I'd envision a seesaw. Let's say that a level seesaw means no depression and whenever either end touches the ground that's depression. One end is genes/physiology; the other is environment. There are some people who are so genetically predisposed to depression that even minor environmental challenges—the types of things that are inescapable in this world—drive them into a depression causing the seesaw to hit the ground. Similarly, there are some environments that are so depressogenic that all but the most resilient of us would become depressed—with the result that the seesaw again hits the ground. In most cases, moderate genetic vulnerability meets fairly rough environments—this is the most common scenario for giving birth to depression in my view.

There is another important point to make here, and that is the fact that the relative contributions of physiology versus environment in the onset of a depressive episode changes with time. Significant data show that the vast majority of first depressive episodes are preceded by events that all of us would recognize as stressful.[6] This is the case with your man in his mid-50s. We can all see why he got depressed. But the physiological processes that give rise to depression appear clearly to damage the brain,[7] such that over time the brain and body become more and more vulnerable to depression, with the result that less and less stress is required to launch a new episode. Some people interpret this pattern as demonstrating that depression becomes autonomous, or freewheeling, with time, and hence truly "organic" in the way that you use the term. I suspect something rather different is the case, and that is that more and more minor stressors are capable of toppling a person's fragile composure. Many of these stressors are idiosyncratic to the individual involved, aren't picked up easily by standardized questionnaires, and hence are missed. By the way, to my knowledge, no one has ever adequately tested which of these two possibilities is closer to the truth.

So, to summarize, our best data suggest that all depressions, no matter how situational, are profoundly organic; and all "organic depressions," no matter how apparently autonomous of environmental conditions, have at the least a history of stress vulnerability that got the depressive process started.

REFERENCES
1. Kendler KS, Karkowski LM, Prescott CA. Causal relationship between stressful life events and the onset of major depression. *Am J Psychiatry*. 1999;156(6):837-841.
2. Kendler KS, Gardner CO. Monozygotic twins discordant for major depression: a preliminary exploration of the role of environmental experiences in the aetiology and course of illness. *Psychol Med*. 2001;31(3):411-423.
3. Kendler KS, Karkowski-Shuman L. Stressful life events and genetic liability to major depression: genetic control of exposure to the environment? *Psychol Med*. 1997;27(3):539-547.
4. Kendler KS. Anna-Monika-Prize paper. Major depression and the environment: a psychiatric genetic perspective. *Pharmacopsychiatry*. 1998;31(1):5-9.
5. Chiao JY, Blizinsky KD. Culture-gene coevolution of individualism-collectivism and the serotonin transporter gene. *Proc Biol Sci*. 2010;277(1681):529-537.
6. Kendler KS, Thornton LM, Gardner CO. Genetic risk, number of previous depressive episodes, and stressful life events in predicting onset of major depression. *Am J Psychiatry*. 2001;158(4):582-586.
7. Frodl TS, Koutsouleris N, Bottlender R, et al. Depression-related variation in brain morphology over 3 years: effects of stress? *Arch Gen Psychiatry*. 2008;65(10):1156-1165.

Bipolar Disorder in Children and Adolescents

QUESTION: "Is bipolar disorder a 'real' condition in children and adolescents? I hear so much controversy surrounding this issue in the press and would appreciate your clarification."

Rakesh Jain, MD, MPH:

If there is one controversial issue in the world of mental health, this is it! The single most controversial issue in psychiatry is articulated in your question, and it deserves close examination from us clinicians.

First of all, it's important to remember that the *Diagnostic and Statistical Manual of Mental Disorders-IV* (*DSM-IV*) does not tell us that there is any age limit to making a diagnosis of bipolar disorder (BD). From the point of view of what our major diagnostic text tells us, there is no prohibition from making the diagnosis in any age group as long as the criteria are met.

Why then this controversy? None of us question if major depression or panic disorder belongs exclusively in the domain of adulthood, then why is there such concern about BD?

This may be for multiple reasons.[1,2] BD has only in the last two decades or so been fully appreciated as a common psychiatric condition in both psychiatrists' and primary care physicians' offices; some years behind major depression achieved such recognition. Could this then be the reason why we are slower to come to the appreciation of BD's existence in individuals under 18 years of age?

I think this may play a role, but my feeling is that a far more common reason for such skepticism regarding pediatric BD is because of different clinical presentations in pediatric and adult patients. This issue is key.

What are some of the differences in pediatric and adult BD presentation in our practices? First, pediatric BD often does not have a cyclical presentation of deregulated mood symptoms, and irritability is commonly the most prominent symptom.[3] While adults, too, can present with ultradian rapid cycling and mixed episode presentations, it appears to be more common in youngsters. To complicate matters, attention-deficit/hyperactivity disorder (ADHD) is unusually common in pediatric BD.[4] These two factors, in my opinion, are the most common reasons for diagnostic confusion regarding pediatric BD.

Now, to address the question of whether there is even such a thing as pediatric BD. The answer appears to be yes, and this is based on very careful work conducted at the Washington University School of Medicine.[3] Their work does support the notion that pediatric BD is a "real" condition. The thing to remember, though, is that this group used a relatively narrow criterion, and many "real life" patients we see in our practices have a much broader range of symptoms.

Perhaps another major reason for our confusion regarding pediatric BD comes from its amazingly frequent overlap with ADHD, yet differences have been documented.[5,6] Again, the Washington University group has examined this and found that, while the overlap is common, there are patients who clearly have BD and not just a "worse" or more severe form of ADHD.[3]

A danger worth pointing out is that BD is both over- and underdiagnosed in clinical practices. In other words, vigilance is called for, and our task is to do our best to make the diagnosis of BD in pediatric patients after careful examination of the current presentation, longitudinal course, as well as family history. A recent article on this topic from Leibenluft is very instructive reading.[7] I would also like to recommend another article that focuses on this issue in the primary care office by Cummings and Fristad.[8]

Happy reading!

There is no question that pediatric BD is "real," but stay tuned as a huge amount of research is coming our way that will shed more light on this issue!

REFERENCES
1. Chang KD. Course and impact of bipolar disorder in young patients. *J Clin Psychiatry*. 2010;71(2):e05.
2. Findling RL. Diagnosis and treatment of bipolar disorder in young patients. *J Clin Psychiatry*. 2009;70(12):e45.
3. Craney JL, Geller B. A prepubertal and early adolescent bipolar disorder-I phenotype: review of phenomenology and longitudinal course. *Bipolar Disord*. 2003;5(4):243-256.
4. Singh T. Pediatric bipolar disorder: diagnostic challenges in identifying symptoms and course of illness. *Psychiatry (Edgmont)*. 2008;5(6):34-42.
5. Frazier JA, Breeze JL, Makris N, et al. Cortical gray matter differences identified by structural magnetic resonance imaging in pediatric bipolar disorder. *Bipolar Disord*. 2005;7(6):555-569.
6. Biederman J, Makris N, Valera EM, et al. Towards further understanding of the co-morbidity between attention deficit hyperactivity disorder and bipolar disorder: a MRI study of brain volumes. *Psychol Med*. 2008;38(7):1045-1056.
7. Leibenluft E. Pediatric bipolar disorder comes of age. *Arch Gen Psychiatry*. 2008;65(10):1122-1124.
8. Cummings CM, Fristad MA. Pediatric bipolar disorder: recognition in primary care. *Curr Opin Pediatr*. 2008;20(5):560-565.

Schizophrenia

QUESTION: "Is schizophrenia really a valid diagnostic entity?"

Jon W. Draud, MS, MD:

Many now view schizophrenia along a continuum with schizoaffective disorder and bipolar spectrum illnesses. Certainly, patients who exhibit psychotic symptoms and are misdiagnosed with schizophrenia suffer major disadvantages in terms of treatment with antipsychotics as first-line agents instead of mood stabilizers. Indeed, families and caregivers are adversely affected as well. Not to be understated is the cost of diagnosing schizophrenia, which was estimated to be $62.7 billion in the United States alone in 2002. Thus, many authors and much research now support the idea that schizophrenia and bipolar affective disorder are more alike than they are different.

The Kraepelinian dichotomy from the 19th century, which separated schizophrenia diagnostically from bipolar affective disorder, is now way obsolete. There are many now who view psychotic illnesses as one disease along a spectrum that encompasses psychotic bipolar (formerly thought of as schizophrenia), bipolar disorder with moderate psychotic signs and symptoms (formerly schizoaffective disorder), and classic bipolar affective disorder (non-psychotic type with prominent mood symptoms).

As clinicians, we know that most patients diagnosed with schizophrenia have prominent mood signs and symptoms—especially depressed mood, and it is extremely rare to see "schizophrenic" patients with no mood symptomatology. In the very small percent of patients who exhibit psychotic symptoms with no mood disturbance, my opinion would be that psychotic disorder NOS may better serve the long-term prognosis than a diagnosis of schizophrenia. The idea being that eventually most of these patients will develop mood symptoms, and if they undergo treatment with antipsychotics too early, the mood symptoms will be mashed and/or exacerbated by the pharmacologic regimen. This can be considered heretical by some; myself and many others believe that there is essentially no such pure diagnostic entity as "schizophrenia."

Cognitive Therapy and Schizophrenia

QUESTION: "In view of the specific structural and neuroendocrine changes now known to occur in schizophrenia, is there *any* role for therapy—such as cognitive therapy or cognitive enhancement therapy?"

Rakesh Jain, MD, MPH:

Your excellent question immediately reveals two issues. First, and you are correct, we now have a tremendous amount of information that establishes schizophrenia's structural and neuroendocrine impact on the patient's brain and body.[1-6] The body's inflammatory chemokine system is also dysregulated, raising concerns about the long-term impact on morbidity and mortality in these patients.[7-9]

The second issue is that, unintentionally, you are revealing a bias many of us suffer from—that if a disorder has a biological "signature" (such as structural and neuroendocrine changes), then a mere "psychological" intervention such as cognitive therapy would have no or diminished role in helping patients.

This bias, which truly is widely held, deserves to be debunked. It is incumbent upon us clinicians to not see cognitive therapy as merely a psychological intervention that could not possibly have an impact on predominantly biological disorders such as schizophrenia. To dispel this bias, we must first closely examine the data at hand regarding cognitive therapy and cognitive enhancement therapy in patients afflicted with schizophrenia.

Let's start this conversation by first acknowledging two salient and well established facts. Schizophrenia does indeed have a well-known, and often replicated, evidence base for structural changes in various parts of the brain, as well as neuroendocrine changes that adversely affect them. Secondly, tremendous strides have been made in the development of antipsychotics, and multiple atypical antipsychotics have recently been introduced, thereby bringing an ever-improving balance between efficacy and tolerability. However, despite these advances, the lives of patients with schizophrenia remain significantly impaired, and bio-psycho-social (all three) interventions are needed for optimized recovery.[10]

Now, let's turn our attention to the evidence at hand regarding cognitive therapy's impact on patients with schizophrenia.

Quite impressively, a recent study found that cognitive enhancement therapy offered gray matter neuroprotection in patients with schizophrenia.[11] In a two-year randomized study, patients participating in cognitive enhancement therapy showed significantly greater preservation of gray matter volume in the left hippocampus, parahippocampal gyrus, and fusiform gyrus, as well as significantly greater gray matter increases in the left amygdala ($P<0.04$) compared with patients participating in enriched supportive therapy. "Less gray matter loss in the left parahippocampal and fusiform gyrus and greater gray matter increases in the left amygdala were significantly related to improved cognition and mediated the beneficial cognitive effects of cognitive enhancement therapy," concluded the study authors.

Now you see why I worry that ignoring nonpharmacologic therapies may be detrimental to our patients' long-term outcomes?

Here's another question we must ask ourselves: Does cognitive therapy offer help with the positive or the negative symptoms of schizophrenia? The answer appears to be—*both*, with data supporting this therapy's salutary effects both the damaging effects of positive[12] and negative symptoms of schizophrenia.[13,14]

Another question to ask: Do cognitive-based therapies help with acute reduction of symptoms or do they help with relapse prevention? The answer appears to be *both*. A recent study revealed that cognitive behaviorally based therapy did indeed significantly reduce relapse rates as compared to treatment as usual.[15] This is one more feather in the cap for add-on cognitive therapy to antipsychotic medications!

Is the combination of antipsychotics with cognitive therapies superior to just antipsychotics alone? The answer, based on empirical studies, appears to be *yes*,[16] thereby adding another weapon to our armamentarium against this savage disease.

Does cognitive therapy have to be individual or could it be effective in a cost-effective group setting? Evidence does show that group-based cognitive therapy was effective.[17] There is even evidence for home-delivered cognitive-based therapies being effective.[18]

A survey of clinical practices reveals that clinicians in the United States appear to have a greater bias against cognitive therapy's usefulness in schizophrenia than our European colleagues.[19] This bias is damaging to our patients, and we must confront it. I encourage you to further read on the issue of nonpharmacologic augmentation of medication treatment in schizophrenia, and I recommend the following review articles for a more detailed examination of cognitive therapies in schizophrenia.[20-23]

In closing, I would like to make the following points:

 — Schizophrenia is indeed a heavily biologically-based disorder, with overwhelming evidence for adverse structural, neuroendocrine, and inflammatory cytokine changes;

 — Antipsychotics, particularly the atypicals, are the standard of care for these patients;

 — Cognitive-based therapies, even though "psychological," demonstrate both psychological and biological improvements in patients with schizophrenia;

 — We North American clinicians appear to be more biased against cognitive-based therapies than our European colleagues; this is an issue we must proactively address; and

 — Cognitive-based therapies appear to be effective in combination therapy with antipsychotics for acute treatment of both positive and negative symptoms, for both acute episodes and relapse prevention, and appear to improve patient quality of life in multiple ways.

REFERENCES

1. Bradley AJ, Dinan TG. A systematic review of hypothalamic-pituitary-adrenal axis function in schizophrenia: implications for mortality. *J Psychopharmacol*. 2010;24(4 Suppl):91-118.
2. Guest PC, Schwarz E, Krishnamurthy D, et al. Altered levels of circulating insulin and other neuroendocrine hormones associated with the onset of schizophrenia. *Psychoneuroendocrinology*. 2011;[Epub ahead of print].
3. Goldman MB, Wang L, Wachi C, et al. Structural pathology underlying neuroendocrine dysfunction in schizophrenia. *Behav Brain Res*. 2011;218(1):106-113.
4. Hempel RJ, Tulen JH, van Beveren NJ, et al. Diurnal cortisol patterns of young male patients with schizophrenia. *Psychiatry Clin Neurosci*. 2010;64(5):548-554.
5. Levitt JJ, Bobrow L, Lucia D, Srinivasan P. A selective review of volumetric and morphometric imaging in schizophrenia. *Curr Top Behav Neurosci*. 2010;4:243-281.
6. McIntosh AM, Owens DC, Moorhead WJ, et al. Longitudinal volume reductions in people at high genetic risk of schizophrenia as they develop psychosis. *Biol Psychiatry*. 2010;[Epub ahead of print].
7. Reale M, Patruno A, De Lutiis MA, et al. Dysregulation of chemo-cytokine production in schizophrenic patients versus healthy controls. *BMC Neurosci*. 2011;12(1):13.
8. Watanabe Y, Someya T, Nawa H. Cytokine hypothesis of schizophrenia pathogenesis: evidence from human studies and animal models. *Psychiatry Clin Neurosci*. 2010;64(3):217-230.
9. Paul-Samojedny M, Kowalczyk M, Suchanek R, et al. Functional polymorphism in the interleukin-6 and interleukin-10 genes in patients with paranoid schizophrenia-a case-control study. *J Mol Neurosci*. 2010;42(1):112-119.
10. Bromley E, Brekke JS. Assessing function and functional outcome in schizophrenia. *Curr Top Behav Neurosci*. 2010;4:3-21.
11. Eack SM, Hogarty GE, Cho RY, et al. Neuroprotective effects of cognitive enhancement therapy against gray matter loss in early schizophrenia: results from a 2-year randomized controlled trial. *Arch Gen Psychiatry*. 2010;67(7):674-682.
12. Erickson DH. Cognitive-behaviour therapy for medication-resistant positive symptoms in early psychosis: a case series. *Early Interv Psychiatry*. 2010;4(3):251-256.
13. Thomas N, Rossell S, Farhall J, Shawyer F, Castle D. Cognitive behavioural therapy for auditory hallucinations: effectiveness and predictors of outcome in a specialist clinic. *Behav Cogn Psychother*. 2011;39(2):129-138.
14. Klingberg S, Wittorf A, Herrlich J, et al. Cognitive behavioural treatment of negative symptoms in schizophrenia patients: study design of the TONES study, feasibility and safety of treatment. *Eur Arch Psychiatry Clin Neurosci*. 2009;259 Suppl 2:S149-S154.
15. Klingberg S, Wittorf A, Fischer A, et al. Evaluation of a cognitive behaviourally oriented service for relapse prevention in schizophrenia. *Acta Psychiatr Scand*. 2010;121(5):340-350.
16. Pinninti NR, Rissmiller DJ, Steer RA. Cognitive-behavioral therapy as an adjunct to second-generation antipsychotics in the treatment of schizophrenia. *Psychiatr Serv*. 2010;61(9):940-943.
17. Bechdolf A, Knost B, Nelson B, et al. Randomized comparison of group cognitive behaviour therapy and group psychoeducation in acute patients with schizophrenia: effects on subjective quality of life. *Aust N Z J Psychiatry*. 2010;44(2):144-150.
18. Velligan DI, Draper M, Stutes D, et al. Multimodal cognitive therapy: combining treatments that bypass cognitive deficits and deal with reasoning and appraisal biases. *Schizophr Bull*. 2009;35(5):884-893.
19. Kuller AM, Ott BD, Goisman RM, Wainwright LD, Rabin RJ. Cognitive behavioral therapy and schizophrenia: a survey of clinical practices and views on efficacy in the United States and United Kingdom. *Community Ment Health J*. 2010;46(1):2-9.
20. Morrison AK. Cognitive behavior therapy for people with schizophrenia. *Psychiatry* (Edgmont). 2009;6(12):32-39.
21. Rathod SP, Phiri P, Kingdon D. Cognitive behavioral therapy for schizophrenia. *Psychiatr Clin North Am*. 2010;33(3):527-536.
22. Tai S, Turkington D. The evolution of cognitive behavior therapy for schizophrenia: current practice and recent developments. *Schizophr Bull*. 2009;35(5):865-873.
23. Tarrier N. Cognitive behavior therapy for schizophrenia and psychosis: current status and future directions. *Clin Schizophr Relat Psychoses*. 2010;4(3):176-184.

Hallucinations in Schizophrenia

QUESTION: "Why do people with schizophrenia experience hallucinations?"

Vladimir Maletic, MS, MD:

Hallucinations are one of the core "positive" symptoms of schizophrenia. They are often described as perceptual experiences without corresponding external or internal sensory stimuli.[1] Although hallucinations in schizophrenia may involve different sensory modalities (auditory, visual, tactile, etc.) our primary focus will be auditory verbal hallucinations (AVH). Approximately 60% to 80% of patients with schizophrenia[2] at some point in their illness "hear voices," making auditory hallucinations one of the most frequent and fundamentally disturbing symptoms. Patients often report hearing words, intrusive disparaging comments, fragments of conversations, multiple voices arguing, and sometimes commands urging them to act. Most often the voices are different than one's own. One in four patients will experience AVHs that are not responsive to medication treatment.[1]

Let us begin our conversation by briefly reviewing the anatomy and physiology of auditory processing. In healthy individuals, highly integrated neural loops process sensory information, assigning it meaning and emotional value, and determining if it is of internal or external origin. For example, auditory signals are conducted from sensory organs (ears) via cochlear nerves, its corresponding nuclei and mesencephalic relay centers to thalamic receptive fields. From there, information is conveyed to the primary auditory cortex (AI) in the Heschl's gyrus of the temporal lobe. Superior temporal lobe and adjacent temporal-parietal junction (including inferior parietal lobe) and inferior frontal gyrus also contain language centers and secondary association zones,[1] allowing spoken word to be incorporated into a wider social communication context. Arcuate fasciculus is a band of white matter forming principal connection between frontal and temporo-parietal language areas.[3] Loops that include connections between auditory cortex and meso-temporal limbic areas (hippocampal-parahippocampal complex) provide for emotional associations and language-based memory. Additionally, cortico-striatal-thalamo-cortical circuitry plays a major role in speech generation, imagery, and perception.[4] Cortico-thalamic-cerebellar circuits are involved in filtering neocortical input and interpretation of inputs.[5]

Despite intensive studies pathophysiology of AVH in schizophrenia is not fully elucidated. There are several confounding issues: a) schizophrenia is probably not a homogeneous diagnostic category; b) auditory hallucinations may have a different character: from simple words to multiple different voices arguing—we cannot assume that these phenomena have the same neurobiological underpinning; c) studies have used different methodologies, including diverse imaging techniques (positron emission tomography [PET], functional magnetic resonance imaging [fMRI], etc.) and different ways of communicating presence of hallucinations; d) patient samples differ in age, illness duration, medication status, gender, and ethnicity, and; e) sample sizes are often quite small.

Functional imaging studies utilized PET and fMRI to evaluate hallucination as a state or a trait. State studies compare brain activity during presence and absence of hallucinations in the same participants; by contrast, trait studies make comparisons between participants with schizophrenia who have suffered from hallucination, ones who have never hallucinated, and healthy controls.[2]

Trait studies. A recent meta-analysis has found decreased activity in left superior and middle temporal lobes in hallucinating patients with schizophrenia compared to participants who had no history of hallucinations (these areas include primary and associative auditory cortices involved in speech perception). Additionally, hallucinating participants also exhibited hypoactivity in inferior frontal gyrus (IFG), an area that incorporates Broca's convolution, involved both in preparation for overt speech and production of inner speech. Lesser activity in anterior cingulate cortex, an area involved in self-monitoring, may reflect a propensity of hallucinating patients to misinterpret their own inner speech as alien.[2]

State studies. Two recent meta-analyses identified increased activation in IFG and adjacent pre-central gyrus (both components of Broca's area) in hallucinating patients. Furthermore, patients with schizophrenia experiencing hallucinations also had greater activity in their inferior parietal lobule (IPL, a part of speech processing Wernicke's area).[1,2] One of the studies also noted elevated activity in right anterior insula, an area that has an analogue role to the left-sided Broca's area. Both are involved in syntactic processing and verbal imagery, lending support to suggestions that impaired language lateralization may be conducive to emergence of AVH. Elevated activity in associative auditory areas in middle and superior temporal gyri also differentiated hallucinating patients from the ones who did not share their state.

Finally, abnormal activity in parahippocampal-hippocampal area was observed in hallucinating patients. Since these areas play a major role in verbal and contextual memory, it is possible that memory related processes may play a role in generating AVH. A rare PET imaging study evaluated brain metabolic changes in unmedicated first-episode schizophrenic patients. In addition to already described temporal lobe changes, this study also noted altered activity in dorsal medial prefrontal cortex (dmPFC) and cerebellum.[5] dmPFC has been previously identified as an area involved in internal self representation. Its dysfunction combined with aberrant cerebellar processing in hallucinating patients may be reflected in misattribution of inner speech as an external event. In summary, it appears that hallucinations may be an outcome of aberrant activation within a distributed neural network involved in perception, generation, and monitoring of speech, and verbal memory related processes.[1,2,5]

Structural studies. Voxel-based analysis utilizing MRI found correlation between severity of auditory hallucinations and structural changes in several cortical areas.[6] Affected areas included superior and middle temporal gyri (including primary and secondary auditory areas), IPL (encompassing Wernicke's speech receptive area), and posterior cingulate cortex (involved in switching from default network resting activity to active attention). Other studies have described abnormal cortical gyrification in chronically hallucinating patients with schizophrenia, pointing to neurodevelopmental predilection to AVH.[1] Findings of structural imaging studies are echoed by pathohistological evidence. Cytological studies of primary auditory and association cortices have discovered diminished volume of pyramidal neurons and reductions of dendritic spines and buttons in the brains of patients suffering from schizophrenia.[7] Previous studies have also noted impaired *prosody* in schizophrenic patients: manifested as difficulty with speech intonation and recognition of the emotional tone of spoken content. Limited capacity to distinguish between questions and statements, sincerity, and sarcasm further impedes social functioning.[7]

Alterations in anatomical and functional connectivity. Arcuate fasciculus is the main connection between frontal and temporo-parietal language areas. Diffusion tensor imaging studies have detected a relationship between disrupted integrity of this white matter bundle and severity of hallucinations in patients with schizophrenia.[3] These imaging findings most likely correspond with altered cytoarchitecture of axons and supportive glia cells. Furthermore, cytological studies have identified dysfunction and reduced numbers of oligodendroglia in patients with schizophrenia.[7] Functional connectivity computed from fMRI data demonstrated robustly greater connectivity in the loop linking ILP-Wernicke's area with IFG-Broca's complex and putamen, distinguishing hallucinating from non-hallucinating patients and healthy controls.[4] It is plausible to conclude that hyperconnectivity within corticostriatal circuitry may not only predispose patients to hallucinations, but also reflect intensity of auditory hallucinatory experiences in individuals with schizophrenia.

Summary of data indicates that aberrant pattern of activity, in distributed language-processing and producing cortical and subcortical areas, may predispose patients with schizophrenia to auditory hallucinations. Convergent data implicate functional, structural, and connectivity alterations in synergistically disrupting language-based neural processing, resulting in confusion and misinterpretation.

REFERENCES

1. Jardri R, Pouchet A, Pins D, Thomas P. Cortical activations during auditory verbal hallucinations in schizophrenia: a coordinate-based meta-analysis. *Am J Psychiatry.* 2011;168(1):73-81.
2. Kuhn S, Gallinat J. Quantitative meta-analysis on state and trait aspects of auditory verbal hallucinations in schizophrenia. *Schizophr Bull.* 2010;[Epub ahead of print].
3. de Weijer AD, Mandl RC, Diederen KM, et al. Microstructural alterations of the arcuate fasciculus in schizophrenia patients with frequent auditory verbal hallucinations. *Schizophr Res.* 2011;[Epub ahead of print].
4. Hoffman RE, Fernandez T, Pittman B, Hampson M. Elevated functional connectivity along a corticostriatal loop and the mechanism of auditory/verbal hallucinations in patients with schizophrenia. *Biol Psychiatry.* 2011;69(5):407-414.
5. Horga G, Parellada E, Lomena F, et al. Differential brain glucose metabolic patterns in antipsychotic-

naïve first-episode schizophrenia with and without auditory verbal hallucinations. *J Psychiatry Neurosci.* 2011;36(1):100085.

6. Nenadic I, Smesny S, Schlosser RG, Sauer H, Gaser C. Auditory hallucinations and brain structure in schizophrenia: voxel-based morphometric study. *Br J Psychiatry.* 2010;196(5):412-413.

7. Lewis DA, Sweet RA. Schizophrenia from a neural circuitry perspective: advancing toward rational pharmacological therapies. *J Clin Invest.* 2009;119(4): 706-716.

Chapter 6

INCORPORATING WELLNESS INTO CLINICAL PRACTICE

Effect of Spirituality on Inflammatory Response and Depression: Part 1

QUESTION: **"What effect does spirituality have on decreasing the inflammatory response and depression?"**

Charles Raison, MD:

I'm glad to get a chance to answer this question because I probably know about as much regarding this topic (or at least the inflammation part of it) as anyone on earth. Based on this expertise, I can assure you that we don't really know the answer! In fact, I suspect there probably isn't a single answer. I'll focus on one answer in this discussion, which focuses on our research on compassion meditation and inflammatory responses to stress. Next, I'll focus on what we know regarding spirituality and depression. But before I do this, let's talk about the issue more generally.

Here is the rub. Spirituality is a very broad term that covers multiple domains. Moreover, from a physical and mental health point of view, there are good and bad types of spirituality. For example, studies have shown that belief in a vindictive God is associated with increased mortality.[1] If you believe in a just and vengeful God, data suggest that you will die sooner than if you believe in a good old guy in the sky, or even in nothing.[1] Consistent with this, many measures of mortality and overall health are worse in the United States, with a high prevalence of fundamentalist Christian religion when compared to more secular states.[2] I could go on…Christian Scientists who don't believe in accepting modern medical treatment die a number of years sooner than the average American[3]…and so on.

On the other hand, there are many studies suggesting that spirituality can enhance multiple measures of health and well-being.[4] In general, the strongest factor mediating this effect appears to be the close social connections fostered by religious affiliation.[5-7] At least some data suggest that beliefs are not irrelevant. For example, somewhat in contradistinction to what I said above, some evidence suggests that fundamentalists in the United States are happier than more liberally minded Christians, and this happiness associates with a firm and concrete conviction that they are heading to a personal afterlife that will blunt the tragedy of death.[8]

A number of studies have looked at various measures of spirituality and inflammation, and the findings are generally in a beneficial direction.[4] Probably the most replicated finding is that participation in an organized religion is associated with lower levels of proinflammatory cytokines—such as interleukin (IL)-6—in the blood.[9,10] An important point to be made is that these studies are cross-sectional. I've never seen a study in which one group was randomized to become religious and another group was randomized to become irreligious, and cytokine levels were measured before and after this intervention. How could it even be done? The problem with cross-sectional studies is that they don't establish causality. Maybe people who are healthier and happier—and hence have less inflammation—feel more like going to church and being around people. You see the problem? Similarly, I've never seen a study looking at the inflammatory correlates of negative types of spirituality, such as I discussed above.

Our research group at Emory has come as close as anyone to doing a longitudinal examination of whether becoming more spiritual reduces inflammation. I want to emphasize that we have only examined one small part of spirituality and only in a small group of young adults. This being said let me describe what we've done and what we've found.

Spirituality is a complex concept. But certainly two of its primary components—found in all religions—are built around relationships: in the first case, one's relationship with a higher power (even if that higher power is a perfected self), and in the second case, one's relationships with other humans. As I've suggested above, most of the health benefit from religion seems to come from its ability to improve the second type of relationships. While people's feelings about God or the Universe or a Higher Power can have both positive and negative effects on well-being, there is no doubt that anything that improves one's relationships with other people is going to be good for health.[11] In the modern world "good for your health" increasingly appears to also mean "reduces inflammation."[12-19]

Based on this line of thinking, my collaborator, Geshe Lobsang Tenzin Negi, and I decided to examine whether Tibetan Buddhist meditation practices designed to radically enhance compassion toward other people might help people better cope with interpersonal stress, both emotionally and physiologically. Our reasoning was simple. Compassion meditation practices teach people to see everyone in one's life and beyond as sources of benefit rather than threat.[20,21] These practices—by inculcating this perspective—are widely held to generate a world view in which all people are viewed with acceptance and caring. We know from other studies that this type of emotional perspective powerfully fosters positive relationships.[22] Positive relationships improve health and promote stress resilience. So compassion meditation should enhance stress resilience.

To test this idea, we randomized 61 Emory University college freshmen to either six weeks of training in a secularized version of compassion meditation (developed by Geshe Lobsang) or to a health discussion control group. After these interventions, all participants underwent a widely used laboratory-based stressor called the Trier Social Stress Test (TSST). The TSST has been repeatedly shown to elicit a classic stress response, as reflected in elevated blood pressure and heart rate and increased production of the classic stress hormone cortisol. More recently, the TSST has been shown to also reliably increase plasma concentrations of IL-6, a major proinflammatory cytokine.[23] Moreover, work from our group at Emory had shown that medically healthy individuals with depression produce significantly more IL-6 in response to the TSST than do medically healthy individuals without depression.[24]

We hypothesized that participants randomized to compassion meditation would show reduced cortisol, IL-6, and distress responses to the TSST, and that within the meditation group, amount of time spent practicing would be correlated with TSST responses (i.e., more practice, lower IL-6, cortisol, and distress reactions).

As often happens in studies, our hypotheses were only partly confirmed (which is why science is more interesting than nursing preconceived ideas). We found no difference between groups randomized to compassion meditation and the health discussion control group on any measure of stress response. On the other hand, within the meditation group we found a strong correlation between increased practice time during the study and reduced IL-6 and distress responses to the TSST. Moreover, when we divided the meditation group into two subgroups based on a median split of practice time, we saw that the "high-practice" meditation group had significantly lower IL-6, heart rate, and distress responses to the stressor than did either the "low-practice" meditation or the control groups.[25]

These findings strongly suggested a link between amount of practice and improved stress responses, but as you might be thinking, leave unanswered an essential causal question. Because we only conducted one TSST after the training, it is possible that participants who came into the study with reduced stress responses might have been more able to practice—thus effectively reversing the arrow of causality. This finding would be interesting (and in keeping with Buddhist views regarding differences in individual predispositions for the spiritual life), but it wouldn't offer much hope in terms of employing compassion meditation to improve mental and physical health.

The obvious solution would be to administer a TSST before and after meditation training to show that increased practice correlates with amount of reduction in stress responses from the first to the second stressor, but this is easier said than done because people have strikingly different tendencies to accommodate to the second stressor.[26] Some people are more freaked out than they were the first time, and some people don't even break a sweat when given a second TSST. In general, people react less to a second TSST, which has made repeating the procedure a challenge.

So before the federal government would give us grant money to do a study with pre- and post-meditation TSSTs, we had to show that we could reliably stress people out twice. This gave us a chance to do two TSSTs in the same people. With this chance came the opportunity to examine whether a TSST given before meditation training predicted how much people practiced. When we did this, we found no correlation whatsoever between any emotional or physiological response to the TSST and how much people subsequently practiced compassion meditation.[27]

Taken together these two studies strongly suggest that engaging in the practice of compassion meditation may reduce emotional and physical responses to stress that are deleterious to emotional and physical health. Whether the same results will be found when we administer a TSST before and after meditation training to the same subjections awaits completion of a large study underway at Emory to address just this question.

So this is a long answer to the first part of your question about the potential of spirituality to reduce inflammation—and particularly inflammatory responses to psychosocial stress that have been shown to be elevated in individuals with depression. This suggests that spirituality—or at least some aspects of it—may protect against depression.

REFERENCES

1. Pargament KI, Koenig HG, Tarakeshwar N, Hahn J. Religious struggle as a predictor of mortality among medically ill elderly patients: a 2-year longitudinal study. *Arch Intern Med.* 2001;161915):1881-1885.
2. Wilkinson R, Pickett K. *The Spirit Level: Why Greater Equality Makes Societies Stronger.* London: Allen Lane; 2009.
3. Simpson WF. Comparative longevity in a college cohort of Christian Scientists. [Published erratum in *JAMA.* 1989;262(21):3000.] *JAMA.* 1989;262(12):1657-1658.
4. Seeman TE, Dubin LF, Seeman M. Religiosity/spirituality and health. A critical review of the evidence for biological pathways. *Am Psychol.* 2003;58(1):53-63.
5. Koenig LB, Vaillant GE. A prospective study of church attendance and health over the lifespan. *Health Psychol.* 2009;28(1):117-124.
6. Gillum RF, King DE, Obisesan TO, Koenig HG. Frequency of attendance at religious services and mortality in a U.S. national cohort. *Ann Epidemiol.* 2008;18(2):124-129.
7. Koenig HG, Hays JC, Larson DB, et al. Does religious attendance prolong survival? A six-year follow-up study of 3,968 older adults. *J Gerontol A Biol Sci Med Sci.* 1999;54(7):M370-M376.
8. Seligman ME. *Authentic Happiness: Using the New Positive Psychology to Realize Your Potential for Lasting Fulfillment.* New York: Free Press; 2002.
9. Ford ES, Loucks EB, Berkman LF. Social integration and concentrations of C-reactive protein among US adults. *Ann Epidemiol.* 2006;16(2):78-84.
10. Koenig HG, Cohen HJ, George LK, et al. Attendance at religious services, interleukin-6, and other biological parameters of immune function in older adults. *Int J Psychiatry Med.* 1997;27(3):233-250.
11. House JS, Landis KR, Umberson D. Social relationships and health. *Science.* 1988;241(4865):540-545.
12. Raison CL, Lin JM, Reeves WC. Association of peripheral inflammatory markers with chronic fatigue in a population-based sample. *Brain Behav Immun.* 2009;23(3):327-337.
13. O'Connor MF, Bower JE, Cho HJ, et al. To assess, to control, to exclude: effects of biobehavioral factors on circulating inflammatory markers. *Brain Behav Immun.* 2009;23(7):887-897.
14. Howren MB, Lamkin DM, Suls J. Associations of depression with C-reactive protein, IL-1, and IL-6: a meta-analysis. *Psychosom Med.* 2009;71(2):171-186.
15. Vidula H, Tian L, Liu K, et al. Biomarkers of inflammation and thrombosis as predictors of near-term mortality in patients with peripheral arterial disease: a cohort study. *Ann Intern Med.* 2008;148(2):85-93.
16. Marsland AL, Gianaros PJ, Abramowitch SM, et al. Interleukin-6 covaries inversely with hippocampal grey matter volume in middle-aged adults. *Biol Psychiatry.* 2008;64(6):484-490.
17. Lampert R, Bremner JD, Su S, et al. Decreased heart rate variability is associated with higher levels of inflammation in middle-aged men. *Am Heart J.* 2008;156(4):759.e1-759.e7.
18. Tan ZS, Beiser AS, Vasan RS, et al. Inflammatory markers and the risk of Alzheimer disease: the Framingham Study. *Neurology.* 2007;68(22):1902-1908.
19. Ridker PM. Inflammatory biomarkers and risks of myocardial infarction, stroke, diabetes, and total mortality: implications for longevity. *Nutr Rev.* 2007;65(12 Pt 2):S253-S259.
20. The Dalai Lama HH. *An Open Heart: Practicing Compassion in Everyday Life.* New York: Little, Brown and Company; 2001.
21. Wallace BA. *Buddhism with an Attitude: The Tibetan Seven-Point Mind Training.* Ithaca, NY: Snow Lion Press; 2008.
22. Lyubomirsky S, King L, Diener E. The benefits of frequent positive affect: does happiness lead to suc-

cess? *Psychol Bull.* 2005;131(6):803-855.

23. Steptoe A, Hamer M, Chida Y. The effect of acute psychological stress on circulating inflammatory factors in humans: a review and meta-analysis. *Brain Behav Immun.* 2007;21(7):901-912.

24. Pace TW, Mletzko TC, Alagbe O, et al. Increased stress-induced inflammatory responses in male patients with major depression and increased early life stress. *Am J Psychiatry.* 2006;163(9):1630-1633.

25. Pace TW, Negi LT, Adame DD, et al. Effect of compassion meditation on neuroendocrine, innate immune and behavioral responses to psychosocial stress. *Psychoneuroendocrinology.* 2009;34(1):87-98.

26. Kirschbaum C, Prussner JC, Stone AA, et al. Persistent high cortisol responses to repeated psychological stress in a subpopulation of healthy men. *Psychosomatic Med.* 1995;57(5):468-474.

27. Pace TW, Negi LT, Sivilli TI, et al. Innate immune, neuroendocrine and behavioral responses to psychosocial stress do not predict subsequent compassion meditation practice time. *Psychoneuroendocrinology.* 2010;35(2):310-315.

Effect of Spirituality on Inflammatory Response and Depression: Part 2

QUESTION: "What effect does spirituality have on decreasing the inflammatory response and depression?"

Charles Raison, MD:

I previously discussed spirituality and inflammation, focusing on research by our group at Emory on the effects of compassion meditation on inflammatory responses to psychosocial stress.[1,2] In this post, we turn to the thornier question of how spirituality relates to depression.

The first thing to say about this issue is that concepts such as "spirituality" and "religion" are very broad and encompass a wide range of emotions, beliefs, and behaviors. Religion has brought us the inquisition and the Dalai Lama.

Given that religion and spirituality have both very bright and very dark faces, it shouldn't be a surprise that taken as a whole they seem to both protect against, and promote, the development of depression.[3] Despite the complications, if one looks through the many studies that have examined this issue, a clear pattern emerges.

The pattern is this: religion as a social factor appears to protect against depression, whereas feelings of intense personal spirituality have a more complex relationship with depression, with some studies showing that inner spirituality may actually be associated with increased rates of depression.[3] Specifically, being involved in an organized religion and attending religious services frequently are associated with reduced rates of depression. However, in a large Canadian study, endorsing that one is a deeply spiritual person predicts increased depressive symptom scores.[4] This finding needs to be balanced against data that people who participate in religion for intrinsic reasons (as opposed to for reasons of self-interest, e.g., business contacts) have lower rates of depression.[5] Also, as noted in my previous post, people who view God as just and vengeful and feel they are, therefore, to one degree or other, spiritual failures are at increased risk of dying.[6]

However, even a factor that is fairly straightforward—like belonging to an organized religion—has wrinkles. Not all religions or denominations appear to be created equal in terms of relationships with depression. As of 1999, for example, data did not support much of a relationship between church attendance and depression in Catholics.[3] On the other hand, members of the Jewish faith appear to have an increased incidence of depression, as do Pentecostals when compared to other conservative Christian groups.[3] People with no religious affiliation are also at increased risk of depression compared to the larger mass of Americans with religious affiliations of one stripe or another.

Disentangling these relationships is the easy part. Much more difficult is to assess which way the arrow of causality is likely to point in all these instances. Is there something in Pentecostalism, for example, that promotes depression in vulnerable parishioners? Does going to church make you feel better and hence less depressed? Does thinking too much about God overwhelm the soul and promote unhappiness? Or are people with depression more likely to be drawn to Pentecostalism, to avoid the social exposure inherent in going to church, and/or to brood about God or turn to the divine as a means of coping with their emotional misery? If I were a betting man, I'd put my money on the second options in general, but there aren't many data to clarify these important considerations.

So far we have discussed spirituality as a form of positive social connection, which is protective against depression, and as a form of inner experience, which seems to be Janus-faced in terms of its relationship with depression: sometimes good, sometimes bad. But spirituality has another face, as reflected in what Jesus said regarding the essence of the Jewish law: "You shall love the Lord, your God, with all your heart, with all your being, with all your strength, and with your entire mind, and your neighbor as yourself." Loving your neighbor as yourself is the essence of compassion, a trait that is powerfully protective against depression.[7]

One can see the protective effects of compassion/altruism by looking at its more mundane manifestations. In this regard, my favorite literature comes from an old mentor of mine at Washington University, C. Robert Cloninger. A leader in personality research, his instrument—the Temperament and Character Inventory (TCI)—assesses three character domains that have spiritual overtones.[8] Self-directedness describes an ability to set long-term goals and to find meaning in life, as well as to listen realistically to positive and negative feedback from others. Cooperativeness describes an ability to get along with and work with others. Self-transcendence more specifically measures feelings and behavior that we would consider spiritual. What I find remarkable is that self-transcendence has been shown to have the same complicated relationship with emotional well-being as is seen with other measures of personal spirituality—whereas individuals high in self-directedness and cooperativeness are remarkably protected from all manner of emotional difficulties.

Self-directedness and cooperativeness describe spirituality in action. Individuals high in these domains live lives organized around higher meanings. They have an ability to listen to and learn from others and an ability to work with others in pursuit of higher goals. This type of life is the ideal of all the major religions, and when put in practice it may be the all-time best preventive for mental disturbance.

REFERENCES

1. Pace TW, Negi LT, Sivilli TI, et al. Innate immune, neuroendocrine and behavioral responses to psychosocial stress do not predict subsequent compassion meditation practice time. *Psychoneuroendocrinology.* 2010;35(2):310-315.
2. Pace TW, Negi LT, Adame DD, et al. Effect of compassion meditation on neuroendocrine, innate immune and behavioral responses to psychosocial stress. *Psychoneuroendocrinology.* 2009;34(1):87-98.
3. McCullough ME, Larson DB. Religion and depression: a review of the literature. *Twin Res.*

1999;2(2):126-136.

4. Baetz M, Griffin R, Bowen R, et al. The association between spiritual and religious involvement and depressive symptoms in a Canadian population. *J Nerv Ment Dis.* 2004;192(12):818-822.

5. Koenig HG, George LK, Peterson BL. Religiosity and remission of depression in medically ill older patients. *Am J Psychiatry.* 1998;155(4):536-542.

6. Pargament KI, Koenig HG, Tarakeshwar N, Hahn J. Religious struggle as a predictor of mortality among medically ill elderly patients: a 2-year longitudinal study. *Arch Intern Med.* 2001;161(15):1881-1885.

7. Steffen PR, Masters KS. Does compassion mediate the intrinsic religion-health relationship? *Ann Behav Med.* 2005;30(3):217-224.

8. Cloninger CR, Svrakic DM, Przybeck TR. A psychobiological model of temperament and character. *Arch Gen Psychiatry.* 1993;50(12):975-990.

Wellness and Depression

QUESTION: "I have been reading about the concept of Wellness. Does this have a role in my practice (I take care of a lot of folks with depression)?"

Rakesh Jain, MD, MPH:

The World Health Organization boldly states that health is *"A state of complete physical, mental and social well-being and not merely the absence of disease or infirmity."*[1] This then raises the obvious questions: Are these lofty and unreasonable goals, or is Wellness a basic human right that all should strive for, regardless of whether they suffer from depression or not?

C. Robert Cloninger, MD, from the Department of Psychiatry of the Washington University School of Medicine recently wrote: *"Psychiatry has failed to improve the average levels of happiness and well-being in the general population, despite vast expenditures on psychotropic drugs and psychotherapy manuals."*[2]

Ouch. That hurts.

While I think Dr. Cloninger is being a bit harsh, there is a large amount of truth in his statement. We clinicians, when treating patients with depression, focus on reducing symptoms and, hopefully, even eliminating them. As the WHO statement above tells us, Wellness is much more than the absence of symptoms; it's the presence of Wellness and well-being too. But in average psychiatry and primary care practices, and in the minds of our patients, this is often not the ultimate goal of treatment.

Other visionary clinicians, too, have weighed in on this topic. Slade[3] recently wrote an article that's boldly titled "Mental Illness and Well-Being: The Central Importance of Positive Psychology and Recovery Approaches." His central theme is that well-being is a need for all, both for those who don't have mental illness, as well as those who do. He has some specific recommendations for us clinicians who wish to incorporate the Wellness model into our practices. He extols us to assess patient's strengths and weaknesses individually, and that the patients' own goals and strengths will guide us into specific Wellness recommendations. He also truthfully acknowledges that the illness model, and not the Wellness model, is the current model of health care delivery around the globe. If we were to accept this new model, significant changes are required in our thinking, treatment plan creation, patients' psychoeducation, and, finally, in societal attitudes toward well-being.

Wellness is not good just for an individual, but also for those around them. For example, in a recent study, children's risk for developmental problems at school entry was found to be related to maternal well-being.[4] Is this positive impact found only in young children? Actually, even in adolescents, a parent's mental well-being strongly and positively impacts the adolescent. A recent study by Giannakopoulos and colleagues[5] revealed that a parent's state of mental well-being impacts their adolescent children's mental and physical well-being. How interesting!

Common sense dictates that this would be the case, but data like this convinces us clinicians to adopt the Wellness model. It's good for our patients, and it's good for those around our patients.

Just from the fact that you asked this question, I suspect you will find a related academic field in psychology of great interest. Positive Psychology, a fairly new but fascinating branch of psychology, has focused on strengths rather than weakness (the traditional model of both psychology and psychiatry, I am unhappy to report), and striking new research shows people can be helped to accept such new models of thinking. This leads to improved well-being. As an introduction to this topic, you may want to check out a book written by the father of positive psychology—Martin E.P. Seligman, PhD—*Authentic Happiness: Using the New Positive Psychology to Realize your Potential for Lasting Fulfillment*. It's a very good primer on the field of positive psychology and the ultimate goal we all strive for—Wellness. It's a book I quite often recommend to my patients who are open to the idea of a higher goal than remission—that of sustained mental well-being.

Well-being absolutely has a role in our practices, no matter what the setting. There are many scales and screeners available for assessment of optimism, well-being, etc., and they are conveniently found on Dr. Seligman's University of Pennsylvania Web Site (www.authentichappiness.sas.upenn.edu/questionnaires. aspx). I encourage you to explore this site; I suspect that you too, just like me, will see many opportunities to bring Wellness into your everyday clinical practice. Your patients will undeniably benefit from this approach.

REFERENCES
1. World Health Organization. *Promoting Mental Health. Concepts, Emerging Evidence, Practice.* Geneva: World Health Organization; 2004.
2. Cloninger CR. The science of well-being: an integrated approach to mental health and its disorders. *World Psychiatry.* 2006;5(2):71-76.
3. Slade M. Mental illness and well-being: the central importance of positive psychology and recovery approaches. *BMC Health Serv Res.* 2010;10:26.
4. Tough SC, Siever JE, Benzies K, et al. Maternal well-being and its association to risk of developmental problems in children at school entry. *BMC Pediatr.* 2010;25(10):19.
5. Giannakopoulos G, Dimitrakaki C, Pedeli X, et al. Adolescents' wellbeing and functioning: relationships with parents' subjective general physical and mental health. *Health Qual Life Outcomes.* 2009;7:100.

Forgiveness

QUESTION: "Can you say more about the role of forgiveness in helping people achieve wellness or optimal mental health? Has the ability and process of forgiving a perpetrator of harm ever been evaluated or studied? As with exercise, I have anecdotally noted improved remission in depression plus posttraumatic stress disorder (PTSD) when a patient is able to feel that forgiveness has taken place. Is anyone looking at this with inflammatory markers or positron emission tomography (PET) scan?"

Charles Raison, MD:

"Peter came to Jesus and asked, 'Lord, how many times shall I forgive my brother when he sins against me? Up to seven times?' Jesus answered, 'I tell you, not seven times, but seventy-seven times [or seventy times seven].'"
Matthew 18:21-22

"All major religious traditions carry basically the same message, that is love, compassion and forgiveness ... the important thing is they should be part of our daily lives."
Dalai Lama

"I forgo all the vengeance in the case of my son [Sonny]...but I'm a superstitious man, and if some unlucky accident should befall him [his other son, Michael], if he should get shot in the head by a police officer, or if he should hang himself in his jail cell, or if he's struck by a bolt of lightning, then I'm going to blame some of the people in this room. And that, I do not forgive."
Don Corleone in The Godfather Part I

Let me start answering this series of important questions by dealing with the easiest one first. Yes, the association between forgiveness and both mental and physical health has been studied repeatedly, and a number of studies have examined whether interventions based on enhancing forgiveness have therapeutic efficacy. To give you a sense of just how much research has been done, go to the computer with me; go to PubMed.gov and type in the word "forgiveness." If you do this, you'll see that 400 peer-reviewed studies have been published since 1990. By way of comparison, only 31 papers on forgiveness were published between 1960 and 1990. So the challenge in answering your other questions lies not in finding information about the relationship between forgiveness and mental or physical health, but rather trying to come to coherent conclusions about what this voluminous literature has to say about this relationship. After having reviewed this literature, it is clear that forgiveness can be good or bad depending on a person's motives and context. Thus, it is too simple to say that learning to always be forgiving is a straightforward pathway to wellness and improved physical health. Rather, as clinicians, the challenge before us is to help our patients see when forgiveness can benefit their well-being and when it can actually cause them harm. Forgiveness can be powerful, but it is no panacea, and should not be proffered by us as being one.

Let's take a closer look.

What is Forgiveness?

Forgiveness is not one thing. Sometimes it can be a freely given gift offered from a position of power. Other times it can be used as a dodge to avoid taking personal responsibility or to face the fact that one is being bullied by someone else. Researchers have defined it as a "prosocial change toward a perceived transgressor,"[1] "a freely made choice to give up revenge, resentment, or harsh judgments toward a person who caused a hurt…and a striving to respond with generosity, compassion, and kindness toward that person."[2,3]

The Good Side of Forgiveness

It is indisputable that forgiveness can be a healing force of good in the world, based both on studies that compare one's ability to forgive with a variety of health outcomes and on studies showing that teaching people to forgive others can improve health and well-being (see below for a discussion of studies examining forgiveness as a therapeutic intervention). In response to your question about PTSD and depression in particular, studies suggest that being able to forgive others is protective against both conditions. A study of 213 veterans with PTSD found that difficulty forgiving oneself and/or others was associated with increased depression, anxiety, and PTSD symptom severity.[4] In a large study of twins, forgiveness and related emotional/behavioral states (e.g., non-vengefulness) were associated with a reduced risk of having either an internalizing or externalizing psychiatric condition.[5] Both a self-forgiving attitude and spirituality were unique predictors of less mood disturbance and better quality of life in women being treated for breast cancer,[6] and forgiveness has been shown to be similarly protective against anxiety and depression in patients with cardiovascular disease.[7] Other studies have shown that an inability to forgive self or others predicts depression, especially in those who hold positive views of forgiveness.[8] One tangible benefit of the positive effect of forgiveness on mood comes in the form of improved sleep in those more able to forgive others.[9]

In addition to protecting against negative emotionality in general and psychiatric disturbance in particular, the ability to forgive has also been associated in a number of studies with improved well-being. One particularly touching example of this comes from a qualitative study done in aged survivors of the atomic bombing of Hiroshima. Those who had responded to the bombing and its aftermath with a life-long tendency toward anxiety and a focus on themselves were found to be "surviving" whereas those who had transcended the catastrophe to thrive (as opposed to merely surviving) were found to demonstrate higher levels of several positive traits, forgiveness among them.[10] People high in emotional intelligence—which is associated with various measures of health and well-being—are less likely than others to hold lasting resentments.[11]

I discuss positive physical effects of forgiveness a little later in this Q&A, but this is an appropriate point to mention an interesting study that found that older adults who were unable to forgive themselves or forgive others, or feel forgiven by God, were more likely to have had an infection in the previous month, although no immune mechanism for this association was tested.[12]

This listing of studies showing health benefits for forgiveness barely scratches the surface of this huge literature and should in no way be seen as presenting all important or interesting findings in this area. But the list is incomplete not just due to brevity, but also to the fact that not all findings regarding forgiveness and health are so rosy, a subject to which we turn now.

The Bad Side of Forgiveness

An essential—and unanswered—question in forgiveness research is whether there can be "too much of a good thing" when it comes to cutting other people a break. If one followed Jesus' advice quoted above and forgave people endlessly, one might achieve the kingdom of heaven, but might not have a viable strategy for living life on this earth. Evidence for this comes from a study that employed a fascinating game called the Prisoner's Dilemma (PD). In PD two individuals interact with each other repeatedly. In each round of the game each player can choose to either cooperate with the other player or "defect." If both players cooperate they each receive a monetary reward, let's say $1. If one defects and one cooperates, the one who defects gets $2 and the one who cooperates gets nothing. Can you guess what happens when both players defect? They each get 50¢.

This game has been studied endlessly because it so obviously captures important truths about interactions with people we have to deal with on a regular basis. Obviously it is best in the long run for the two individuals to develop enough trust in each other so that they cooperate on every turn. But if you are playing with someone who has a penchant for taking advantage of nice people, you will go broke always cooperating, essentially forgiving the other player his or her repeated attempts to take advantage of you. When people can't find a way to cooperate they both lose, but not as much as a player who insists on being cooperative even when the other player doesn't reciprocate. Recent research suggests something even more ominous. Players who always cooperate, regardless of the response of the other player, actually promote the development of defection in the game-mates. Without intending to, they bring out the worst in other people.[13]

These findings may help explain what seems to me to be the darkest side of forgiveness, which is that—as in the PD game—unexamined forgiveness can actually make the world a worse place for the person who forgives too easily and frequently, and for those who are forgiven. For example, a study that followed young adults through the first years of their marriages found that a tendency to easily forgive one's partner early in the relationship was associated with increased psychological and physiological aggression from partner over time; whereas withholding forgiveness actually seemed to make the errant marriage partner behave better over time.[14] How much resentment and flat-out hatred this type of hard-nosed approach generated was not investigated. But here again the prisoner's dilemma suggests something disturbing. One might be able to force a partner to behave better by withholding forgiveness, but this type of strategy—known as "tit-for-tat" in the PD game, makes the emergence of long-term cooperation between players very difficult to achieve.[13]

Another study of forgiveness early in marriage really helps clarify whether forgiving one's partner will lead to one feeling better or worse about oneself as time passes.[15] It turns out that the key factor in whether one's self-respect goes up or down is how the spouse responds to having transgressed in the first place. If the partner works hard to make amends and is an agreeable person who can signal that one will be safe and valued in the relationship moving forward, then the ability to forgive bolsters self-esteem and obviously helps the relationship. If the spouse interprets one's forgiveness as a sign of weakness and takes advantage of it, one is likely to feel more and more like a "doormat" (which is actually in the title of this study) with all the loss of self-worth and esteem that this entails.

But again, there is a complication. A very large, recent study found that people who endorse using this type of "conditional forgiveness" in their daily lives are at increased risk of death from all sorts of natural causes than are those who forgive more and less often.[2]

Finally, although self-acceptance and forgiveness are hot therapeutic topics and often seen to be unqualified goods, a recent study suggests that forgiving oneself too easily carries its own disadvantages. This study found a strong relationship between the degree to which people forgave themselves for failing to quit smoking and their actual ability to quit. The more people forgave themselves, the less likely they were to be able to kick the habit.[16]

What Predicts Forgiveness?

Forgiveness always occurs in a context that includes the person doing the forgiving and the person or people toward whom the forgiveness is directed. As you might expect, the likelihood that forgiveness will occur depends on the character and circumstances of the person doing the forgiving and the context in which the forgiving must occur.[17]

We've already mentioned one factor that greatly increases the likelihood that forgiveness will bring forth emotional well-being, and that is the character and behavior of the person who has done the transgression. The same behavioral and characterological factors also greatly influence whether forgiveness will occur in the first place. Said simply, people are far more likely to forgive someone who is agreeable in general, who apologizes sincerely, and who demonstrates a willingness to make amends.[17] People are also more likely to forgive someone with whom they have a close and committed relationship, especially if the relationship is emotionally satisfying.[17]

Regardless of the situation, some people are more likely to forgive than others. What predicts this? We've already mentioned several of these factors as the fruits of forgiveness (see above), but they also seem to promote a tendency to forgive. Factors associated with being more forgiving include being an empathetic and agreeable person, having high emotional intelligence, being able to see things from others' point of view, and being in a position of power in the relationship that requires forgiveness.[17,18] On the other hand, people who are depressed, angry, or neurotic are less likely than others to forgive.[17] People who are hypercompetitive have trouble forgiving, whereas those with a more balanced sense of competition driven by a desire for personal development are actually more likely than people without this trait to forgive others.[19] Finally, you would think that people with a strong need to have a sense of belonging would be especially likely to forgive, but, in fact, the opposite is the case.[20]

Health and Neurobiology of Forgiveness

Most studies examining health-relevant physiological effects of forgiveness have focused on cardiovascular measures. The news here is good. Multiple studies suggest that forgiveness lowers blood pressure and heart rate and, in general, protects the vascular endothelium from the damaging consequences of psychological stress.[21] Forgiveness appears to proffer these benefits primarily through its ability to protect against depressed moods.

Surprisingly, we know a good deal less about how forgiveness affects brain functioning, and nothing—to my knowledge—about how and if it affects brain structure. In terms of brain functioning, forgiveness seems to require activation of a number of brain areas known to be important for sense of self, as well as the ability to accurately recognize the subjectivity and emotional experiences of other people. Often referred to as the "default mode network," these areas are located in midline cortical and subcortical areas that tend to be more active when people are "thinking about nothing in particular" (meaning that they are usually thinking about themselves in one way or other) and that have been repeatedly implicated in the pathophysiology of depression.[22]

Because my area of research focuses on brain—immune system interactions, I searched diligently to identify studies that had examined the effects of forgiveness on immune or inflammatory functioning, and found none that addressed this issue specifically. Perhaps the closest work I know of comes from our research group. We have spent several years studying the immune effects of a contemplative practice derived from Tibetan Buddhism known as compassion meditation. Practicing acceptance and forgiveness of others is an important part of the practice. Interestingly, we have shown that people who learn and practice compassion meditation have reduced inflammatory and autonomic responses to a laboratory psychosocial stressor, and reduced cortisol and CRP (C-reactive protein; an inflammatory marker) at rest, although these changes were not associated with self-reported increases in ability to forgive others.[23,24]

Therapeutic Potential of Forgiveness

If forgiveness appears, overall, to promote emotional well-being and physical health, one might predict that teaching people to be more forgiving might be of benefit, and this appears to be the case.[17] Of direct relevance to your question about forgiveness and PTSD, a recent study found that when compared to a treatment comprised of anger validation and assertiveness/interpersonal skill building training, forgiveness therapy resulted in significantly greater improvements in depression, anxiety, post-traumatic stress symptoms, and self-esteem in women who had suffered long-term emotional abuse from a partner.[25] Forgiveness interventions have also been shown to reduce myocardial perfusion defects in response to stress,[26] and to help patients with substance abuse histories to maintain sobriety.[27] Interestingly, despite the traditional association of forgiveness with religious practices, secular forgiveness interventions have been reported to be more effective than explicitly religious/spiritual assumptions and principles.[5]

Forgiveness as a Wellness Strategy: One Size Does Not Fit All

If one theme emerges from the information we have provided it is this: forgiveness appears to have huge potential benefits for health, but it is not something that should be prescribed or applied blindly as an unmitigated good for all who come to us for aid. Most people are likely to benefit immensely from learning to be more accepting of others and more forgiving of those who anger them and/or do them wrong. But it is just as true that many other people use forgiveness as a way of avoiding difficult, but necessary, confrontations with those who are abusing or taking advantage of themselves. Being unforgiving of the self is a recipe for despair and depression, but being overly slack on one's weaknesses can lead to various forms of behavioral stasis that can poison the mind and the body.

I think there are two bottom lines here. First, each patient or client must be assessed in terms of his or her unique personality and social situation, prior to making any type of blanket prescriptions in regards to forgiveness as a wellness strategy. Second, what really seems to matter about forgiveness in terms of health benefits is the internal state it produces when it is done right. And by done right, I mean, when it arises from a position of internal strength and well-being that allows one to be less angry at others, while at the same time, not allowing them to take advantage or behave in inappropriate ways towards oneself. This type of forgiveness does not make one a push-over, and does not always mean that relationships will be re-established after major transgressions. It only means that one will make these types of choices from a more rational and empathic internal state that is less likely to bring misery and illness to oneself. When appropriate, this is the type of forgiveness we should help our patients learn to cultivate.

REFERENCES

1. McCullough ME, Pargament KI, Thoresen CE. The psychology of forgiveness: history, conceptual issues, and overview. In: McCullough ME, Pargament KI, Thoresen CE, eds. *Forgiveness: Theory, Research and Practice*. New York: Guilford Press; 2000:1-14.
2. Toussaint LL, Owen AD, Cheadle A. Forgive to Live: Forgiveness, Health, and Longevity. *J Behav Med*. 2011;[Epub ahead of print].
3. Enright RD, Freedman S, Rique J. The psychology of interpersonal forgiveness. In: Enright RD, North J, eds. *Exploring Forgiveness*. Wisconsin: Wisconsin University Press; 1998:46-62.
4. Witvliet CV, Phipps KA, Feldman ME, Beckham JC. Posttraumatic mental and physical health correlates of forgiveness and religious coping in military veterans. *J Trauma Stress*. 2004;17(3):269-273.
5. Kendler KS, Liu XQ, Gardner CO, et al. Dimensions of religiosity and their relationship to lifetime psychiatric and substance abuse. *Am J Psychiatry*. 2003;160(3):496-503.
6. Romero C, Friedman LC, Kalidas M, et al. Self-forgiveness, spirituality, and psychological adjustment in women with breast cancer. *J Behav Med*. 2006;29(1):29-36.
7. Friedberg JP, Suchday S, Srinivas VS. Relationship between forgiveness and psychological and psychological indices in cardiac patients. *Int J Behav Med*. 2009;16(3):205-211.
8. Brown RP. Measuring individual differences in the tendency to forgive: construct validity and links with depression. *Pers Soc Psychol Bull*. 2003;29(6):759-771.
9. Stoia-Caraballo R, Rye MS, Pan W, et al. Negative affect and anger rumination as mediators between forgiveness and sleep quality. *J Behav Med*. 2008;31(6):478-488.
10. Knowles A. Resilience among Japanese atomic bomb survivors. *Int Nurs Rev*. 2011;58(1):54-60.
11. Carvalho D, Neto F, Mavroveli S. Trait emotional intelligence and disposition for forgiveness. *Psychol Rep*. 2010;107(2):526-534.
12. Callen BL, Mefford L, Groer M, Thomas SP. Relationships Among Stress, Infectious Illness, and Religiousness/Spirituality in Community-Dwelling Older Adults. *Res Gerontol Nurs*. 2010;1-12.
13. Imhof LA, Nowak MA. Stochastic evolutionary dynamics of direct reciprocity. *Proc Biol Sci*. 2010;277(1680):463-468.
14. McNulty JK. The dark side of forgiveness: the tendency to forgive predicts continued psychological and physical aggression in marriage. *Pers Soc Psychol Bull*. 2011;37(6):770-783.
15. Luchies LB, Finkel EJ, McNulty JK, Kumashiro M. The doormat effect: when forgiving erodes self-respect and self-concept clarity. *J Pers Soc Psychol*. 2010;98(5):734-749.
16. Wohl MJ, Thompson A. A dark side to self-forgiveness: forgiving the self and its association with chronic unhealthy behaviour. *Br J Soc Psychol*. 2011;50(Pt 2):354-364.
17. Fehr R, Gelfand MJ, Nag M. The road to forgiveness: a meta-analytic synthesis of its situational and dispositional correlates. *Psychol Bull*. 2010;136(5):894-914.
18. Karremans JC, Smith PK. Having the power to forgive: when the experience of power increases interpersonal forgiveness. *Pers Soc Psychol Bull*. 2010;36(8):1010-1023.
19. Collier SA, Ryckman RM, Thornton B, Gold JA. Competitive personality attitudes and forgiveness of others. *J Psychol*. 2010;144(6):535-543.
20. Barnes CD, Carvallo M, Brown RP, Osterman L. Forgiveness and the need to belong. *Pers Soc Psychol Bull*. 2010;36(9):1148-1160.
21. Whited MC, Wheat AL, Larkin KT. The influence of forgiveness and apology on cardiovascular reactivity and recovery in response to mental stress. *J Behav Med*. 2010;33(4):293-304.
22. Farrow TF, Zheng Y, Wilkinson ID, et al. Investigating the functional anatomy of empathy and forgiveness. *Neuroreport*. 2001;12(11):2433-2438.
23. Pace TW, Negi LT, Adame DD, et al. Effect of compassion meditation on neuroendocrine, innate immune and behavioral responses to psychosocial stress. *Psychoneuroendocrinology*. 2009;34(1):87-98.
24. Pace TW, Negi LT, Sivilli TI, et al. Innate immune, neuroendocrine and behavioral responses to psychosocial stress do not predict subsequent compassion meditation practice time. *Psychoneuroendocrinology*. 2010;35(2):310-315.
25. Reed GL, Enright RD. The effects of forgiveness therapy on depression, anxiety, and posttraumatic stress for women after spousal emotional abuse. *J Consult Clin Psychol*. 2006;74(5):920-929.
26. Waltman MA, Russell DC, Coyle CT, et al. The effects of forgiveness intervention on patients with coronary artery disease. *Psychol Health*. 2009;24(1):11-27.
27. Lin WF, Mack D, Enright RD, Krahn D, Baskin TW. Effects of forgiveness therapy on anger, mood, and vulnerability to substance use among inpatient substance-dependent clients. *J Consult Clin Psychol*. 2004;72(6):1114-1121.

about the authors

JON W. DRAUD, MS, MD

Medical Director of Psychiatry, Addiction Medicine Services, Baptist Hospital, Nashville, TN, and Middle Tennessee Medical Center, Murfreesboro, TN; Private Practice, Adult and Adolescent Psychiatry

Dr. Jon W. Draud received his MS in Pharmacology and his MD at the University of Kentucky in Lexington. He received postgraduate medical education at Vanderbilt University Medical Center in Nashville, where he completed a residency in Psychiatry. A Diplomate of the American Board of Psychiatry and Neurology, Dr. Draud is a member of the American Psychiatric Association, American Medical Association, American Academy of Psychiatry and Law, and American Academy of Sleep Medicine. He is active in teaching medical students and residents, and he has delivered over 3,500 professional lectures to medical personnel. Dr. Draud serves on numerous advisory boards, is an active national-level speaker for several companies, and is involved in neurobiological initiatives related to psychiatric illness.

Dr. Draud has been involved in the design and implementation of several neurobiology projects, including the disease states of depression, bipolar disorder, insomnia, and pain, with an emphasis on fibromyalgia and neuropathic pain. Most recently, he was appointed by the MJ Consulting Group to its Neuroscience Advisory Council and is one of the four founding members of the Integrative Neurobiology Educational Institute, which is a nationally based "think tank," aimed at raising public awareness about the neurobiological underpinnings common among many psychiatric disease states.

RAKESH JAIN, MD, MPH

Director of Psychiatric Drug Research, R/D Clinical Research Center, Lake Jackson, TX; Associate Clinical Professor, Department of Psychiatry and Behavioral Sciences, University of Texas Medical School at Houston, Houston, TX.

Dr. Rakesh Jain attended medical school at the University of Calcutta in India, and then attended graduate school at the University of Texas School of Public Health in Houston where he was awarded the National Institute/Center for Disease Control Competitive Traineeship. He graduated from the School of Public Health in 1987 with a Masters of Public Health degree.

Saundra Jain M A PSyD LPc

After graduate school, he was a Postdoctoral Fellow in Research Psychiatry, under the Gerontology Center of the University of Texas Mental Sciences Institute in Houston where he was a recipient of a National Research Service Award for the support of the Post Doctoral Fellowship. After this, he served a three-year residency in Psychiatry at the Department of Psychiatry and Behavioral Sciences at the University of Texas Medical School at Houston, and two years of Child and Adolescent Psychiatry Fellowship.

Dr. Jain is currently involved in multiple research projects studying the effects of medications on short-term and long-term treatment of depression, anxiety, pain/mood overlap disorders, and psychosis in adult and child/adolescent populations. He is also the author of several articles on the issue of mood and pain conditions. He was recently named "Public Citizen of the Year" by the National Association of Social Workers, Gulf Coast Chapter, in recognition of community and peer education and championing of mental health issues.

VLADIMIR MALETIC, MS, MD

Clinical Professor of Neuropsychiatry and Behavioral Science, University of South Carolina School of Medicine, Columbia, SC; Consulting Associate, Division of Child and Adolescent Psychiatry, Department of Psychiatry, Duke University, Durham, NC

Dr. Vladimir Maletic is Clinical Professor of Neuropsychiatry and Behavioral Science at the University of South Carolina School of Medicine in Columbia, and Consulting Associate in the Division of Child and Adolescent Psychiatry in the Department of Psychiatry at Duke University in Durham, North Carolina. Dr. Maletic received his MD in 1981 and his MS in Neurobiology in 1985, both at the University of Belgrade in Yugoslavia. He went on to serve a residency in Psychiatry at the Medical College of Wisconsin in Milwaukee, followed by a residency in Child Psychiatry at Duke University.

Dr. Maletic is a member of several professional organizations, including the Southern Psychiatric Association and American College of Psychiatrists. In addition, he has published numerous articles and has participated in various national and international meetings and congresses. His special areas of interest include neurobiology of mood disorders, pain, anxiety disorders, ADHD, and regulation of sleep and wakefulness. Dr. Maletic is board-certified by the American Board of Psychiatry and Neurology.

CHARLES RAISON, MD

Associate Professor, Clinical Director of the Mind-Body Program, Department of Psychiatry and Behavioral Sciences, Emory University School of Medicine, Atlanta, GA; CNNHealth Mental Health Expert and Mind-Body Consultant; Scientific President, European Association of Clinical Psychoneuroimmunology

Dr. Charles Raison is an associate professor in the Department of Psychiatry and Behavioral Sciences, Emory University School of Medicine. He also serves as Clinical Director of the Mind-Body program at the University. Dr. Raison received his medical degree from Washington University in St. Louis, MO, where he was elected to Alpha Omega Alpha and won the Missouri State Medical Association Award. He completed residency training at the UCLA Neuropsychiatric Institute and Hospital in Los Angeles. Dr. Raison served as Director of Emergency Psychiatric Services and Associate Director of Consultation and Evaluation Services at UCLA prior to joining the faculty at Emory University. The recipient of several teaching awards, Dr. Raison receives research funding from the National Institute of Mental Health, National Center for Complementary and Alternative Medicine, the Centers for Disease Control and Prevention, and the Georgia Department of Human Services. His research focuses on bi-directional relationships between stress and immune systems, as these relate to the development of depression. His research ranges from immune system effects on central nervous system functioning to the application of compassion meditation as a strategy to reduce inflammatory responses to psychosocial stress. In addition to his activities at Emory, Dr. Raison is the mental health expert and Mind-Body Correspondent for cnn.com, serves as Chief Scientific Advisor for Contemplativehealth.com, and is on the editorial board of *Brain, Behavior and Immunity*. He is also Scientific President, European Association of Clinical Psychoneuroimmunology.

about the publisher

CME LLC is a provider of medical education that promotes the ongoing endeavor to narrow the competency and performance gaps that exist within healthcare professionals through convenient, impactful lifelong learning opportunities. Founded in 1978 with the vision to provide high-quality, practical medical education and information for mental health clinicians, CME LLC's reach now expands to educational offerings for primary care, oncology, pain management, and practice management professionals. Among CME LLC's educational offerings is the annual *U.S. Psychiatric and Mental Health Congress*, one of the largest mental health CME meetings in the United States, and the *Treating the Whole Patient* initiatives.

Made in the USA
Lexington, KY
15 November 2011